Also by Daniel Stih

Healthy Living Spaces
Top 10 Hazards Affecting Your Health

Mold Money
How to Save Thousands of Dollars on Mold
Remediation and Make Sure the Mold is Gone

How to Build a Healthy Home
And Prevent the Negative Impacts on Your Health
That Can Result from Poorly Executed Green
Building Initiatives

Unplugged
How to Find and Get Rid of EMFs in Your Home

What Your Builder Should Know

Best Practices for

Building a Healthy Home

Disclaimer

Every building has unique circumstances for which additional specifications or modifications of the information presented here may be required. Readers should hire an architect and builder and contact Healthy Living Spaces® to review their specifications. How applicable and complete the ideas and suggestions in this book are for your project may depend on climate, local building codes, and type of construction. The author does not assume responsibility for actions based on reading this book. The suggestions may be incomplete or inappropriate for your project.

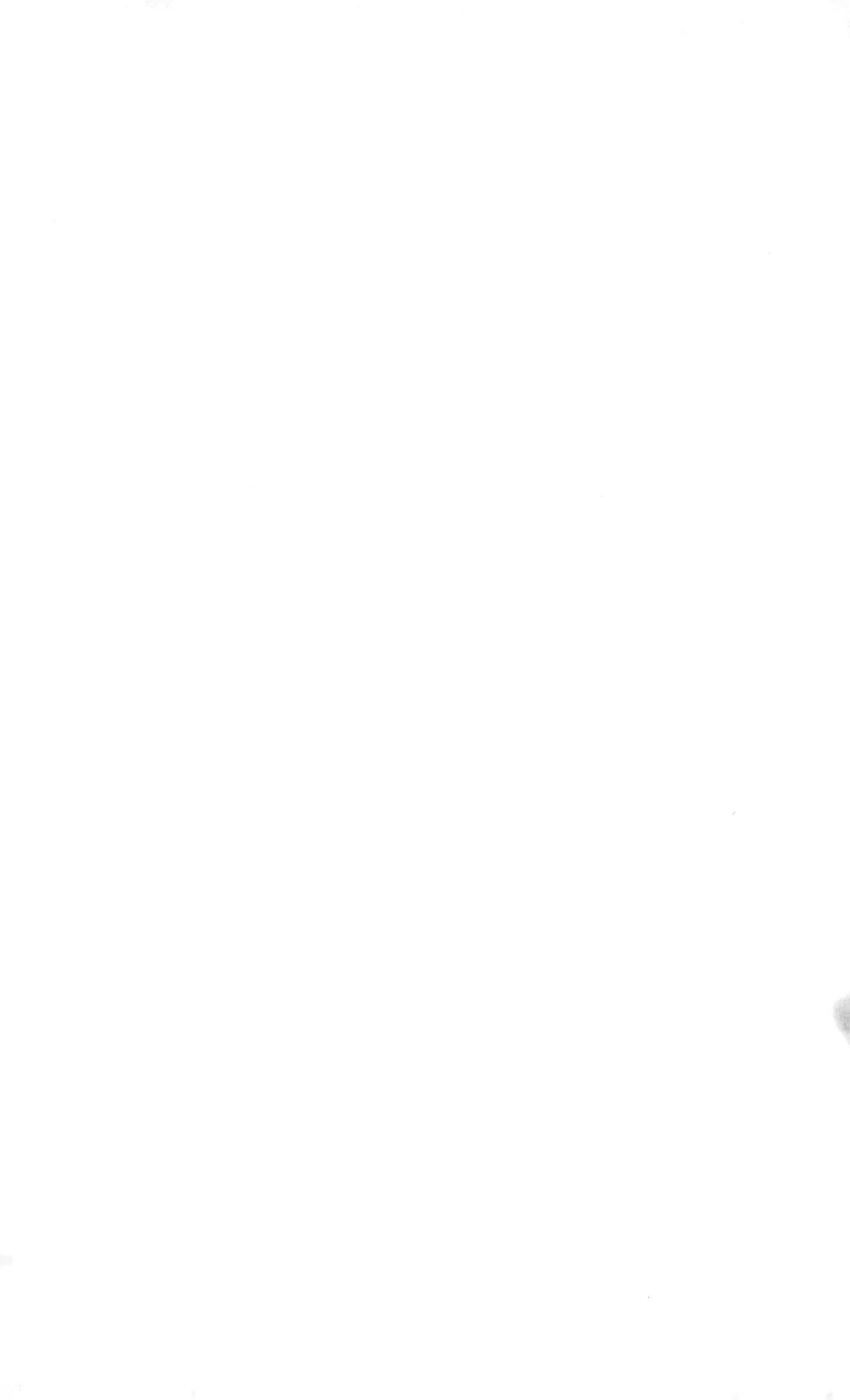

TABLE OF CONTENTS

Introduction

Categories of Concern

Step by Step

The Top 10 Lists

Specifications by Category

Appendix

Introduction

If you are reading this book, chances are you are thinking about building your own home. Congratulations! Building a home is exciting. It can also be challenging. It's more complex to build a residential home than a commercial building. There are numerous choices to be made regarding everything from the type of wood to the color of paint. I wrote this book to make it easy for you. This book explains the most important items that need to be considered when building a healthy home.

This book is a companion to *How to Build a Healthy Home: And Prevent the Negative Impacts on Your Health That Can Result from Poorly Executed Green Building Initiatives*. Whereas the book you are reading is intended to be an easy read, the other contains detailed explanation, charts, and graphs from testing I've performed. It explains how I came to make conclusions about which methods and materials are the healthiest.

It's been a long road here from Aerospace Engineering. After eleven years at a large corporation, I quit my job, moved to a small town, and as fate had it, I became a handyman. I had so much work that I didn't know what to do with it until one day I found myself sick and tired. My doctor said it was from the work I was doing. I was skeptical. When I did not start to feel better, I tried to find healthier ways of building and remodeling.

The door opened to my new career at a store selling non-toxic paint. At the counter was a brochure for courses on how to test the air in homes. The owner put them there, hoping someone would start a business testing homes and refer homeowners to his store for solutions. Other than finding a healthy paint, I didn't make progress finding healthier building materials. I found the testing equipment interesting and spent a small fortune testing every building whose owner let me. My first book, *Healthy Living Spaces: Top 10 Hazards Affecting Your Health,* is based on testing buildings that were causing people to be sick and the solutions I found to make them better.

Through my testing, I discovered that assumptions regarding what's healthy can be wrong. Some materials thought to be unhealthy are not that bad for you; other materials, including those promoted as green, cause health and air quality problems.

This book is written for what is referred to as conventional construction. If you want to build a house using alternative materials—straw bale, rammed earth, pumice, or stone, this book may be used. The interior walls, roof, plumbing, slab, and so forth of buildings are similar.

Because I do not believe a building must be built with natural materials or be green to be healthy, I have been accused of not caring about the environment. I care deeply. When I was a handyman, I frequently went to Habitat for Humanity to look for materials to use and to drop off used materials for them to sell. I saw they were throwing a lot of recyclable materials into the trash. This was in the 1990s, before there were recycling pick-ups for businesses. I offered to help. Habitat agreed to put materials that could be recycled aside and hold them for me to pick up.

The routine was this: the day before trash pickup in my neighborhood, I went to Habitat and picked up the recyclable materials they were saving. Late that night, after stuffing my own recycle bins full, I drove around the neighborhood and unloaded the remainder of the materials into the neighbor's bins I found empty. A neighbor called the police.

Most of us live in conventionally built homes. These can be as healthy as, or healthier than, any type of construction. How you build a house is as much a factor as what you use to build it. As you read the recommendations in this book, consider the cost of following them, your health, and your budget. While it can be hard to build a perfect house, I believe that you will find a few key changes can result in your house being the healthiest in the neighborhood.

What Won't Fix an Unhealthy House

Ozone

Ozone, ionizers, and similar technologies make things worse. There are new chemicals created by the reactions that occur between ozone, the materials a house is built with, and its contents. Chemicals on the surface of materials are rearranged, fragmented, and oxidized into ones more irritating and hazardous than those the treatments are intended to neutralize. For every 100 molecules of ozone that react with pinene, a common fragrance, 15 molecules of formaldehyde are formed. Formaldehyde is created when ozone reacts with the terpenes naturally present in wood. There is an unhealthy outcome when ozone reacts with carpet, paint, heating and air conditioning ducts, and air filters[1].

Bake-out

Bake-out refers to heating a house to increase the rate

new materials off-gas. The idea is if you can make it hot inside a house, the odors will go away quicker. This doesn't work.

Unless ventilation is provided to flush the house with fresh outdoor air at the same time the house is heated, chemicals that off-gas are re-absorbed by other materials in the home. It's difficult to increase the temperate in a home and ventilate it with fresh outdoor air at the same time. The process is ineffective at best. In worst cases it creates new odors and damages materials. A wood floor, for example, should be allowed to acclimatize to prevent shrinking and cracking. The idea that baking a house will fix an air quality problem is a myth.

....

(1) *Organic Indoor Air Pollutants. Occurrence, Measurement, Evaluation.* Edited by Tunga Salthammer and Erick Uhd. Wiley-VCH, 2009. 306.

How to Use This Book

There is a chapter for each step of construction. Each step contains the following:

What It Is

This is a brief description of what occurs during the step.

Categories of Concern

These are the categories of concern. There appears to be three common concerns: mold, ventilation (to clear the air), and reducing electromagnetic fields (EMFs).

Shortcuts and Standard Practices

These are things the average homeowner would never know, capitalized on by builders who do not care how healthy a house is if they can finish it faster. These shortcuts and standard practices are self-defeating for those wanting a healthy home.

What Can Go Wrong Here

These are the common things that can go wrong.

Alternatives

You have choices. This section lists the common options. You may decide to go with what's normal based on cost. An example is air ducts. Furnaces and air-conditioners normally have what are called flex-ducts, ducts made of a flexible, plastic-jacketed material. The plastic off-gases, and the dusts are impossible to clean. The alternative is to use sheet metal for ductwork. Using metal for ductwork adds thousands of dollars to the cost. You might decide you're more concerned about mold, and since it's a dust, not mold issue, you are OK with using flex-ducts.

Recommendations

These are the bare bones, minimum recommendations required to build a healthy home. If you want to do or use something different, substitute what you prefer for what is written in the section "Give This to Your Builder."

How to Use This Book

Check for This

These are the key times to check the builder's work. It may be helpful to hire a general home inspector to go with you. The key items to check are recapped at the end of this book for quick reference.

Give This to Your Builder

The end of each chapter contains specifications that may be handed to a builder. These are formatted according to the Master Format developed by the Construction Specifications Institute. Not everything may apply to your categories of concern. You may want to copy only parts.

This book contains a final section, "Specifications Based on Category." If you are only interested in preventing mold, give the chapter "Specifications for Preventing Mold" to your builder. If you are only interested in EMFs, give the builder "Specifications for Reducing EMFs." Or copy everything at the end of each chapter and give it all to your builder.

Categories of Concern

This section explains why homes are not as healthy as they should be and the known health issues associated with construction practices and materials. Try not to be overwhelmed. You have in your hands a tool to build a healthy home. When you are finished you will have a set of specifications to give the builder.

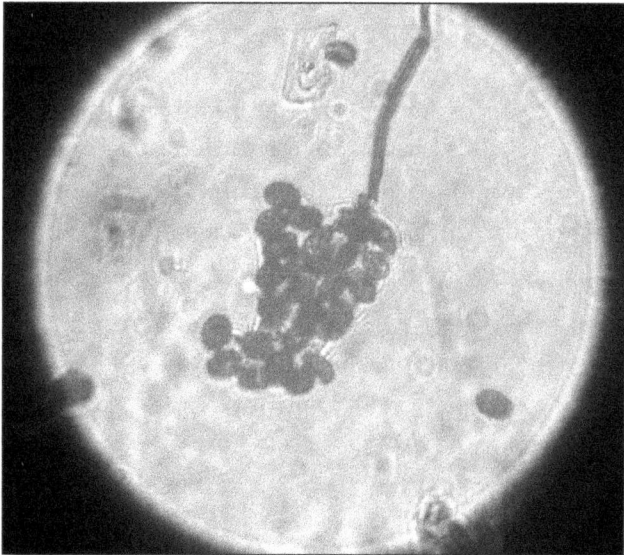

Stachybotrys type mold with spores attached to the hyphae.

Mold

What Is It?

Mold, mildew, and fungus refer to the same thing—the Kingdom of Fungi. If something gets wet and stays wet, mold will grow, no matter how hard you try to stop it. Antimicrobials do not prevent mold for two reasons. There's no product to prevent or kill every type of microorganism; only the surface is affected.

Mold does not grow as soon as something gets wet. Like a seed, spores have an innate intelligence to know when there is enough moisture to germinate. A spore doesn't want to sprout to life at the first sign of moisture, only to dry out a few days later. The average time a material must be wet for mold to grow varies. Depending on the species of mold, a minimum of three days is required.

In its first stage of growth, mold grows roots. These are called mycelium or hyphae. Mold likes water. It is more likely to grow shallow roots in a spider pattern on a surface than to go deep into a material where it is dry. In terms of remediation, the surface on a material such as wood may be cleaned using a wire-brush or sanding. If mold grows into a porous material, such the paper backing on drywall, the material needs to be removed.

Molds do not have stomachs. Molds secrete enzymes that break a material down into simple sugars. The roots absorb the sugars. It's a stinky process. Metabolites are produced that saturate materials and make them smell moldy. The compounds responsible for the odors are called microbial volatile organic compounds (MVOCs) and can cause health symptoms.

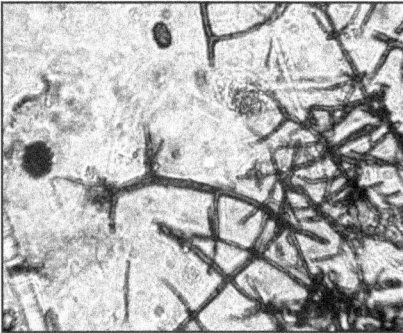

Mycelium and hyphae fragments. A spore of *Stachybotrys* is visible in the upper center. A clump of *Aspergillus* is visible on the left.

Once mold has enough food to support basic life functions, it may produce mycotoxins. The toxins are solids, not gases. They are substances a mold secretes and slathers itself with to protect it from other organisms. The entire fungal structure is coated—spores and mycelium.

Every mold is capable of producing mycotoxins. As it requires energy to produce them, a mold won't produce toxins unless it is required for survival. The type of mycotoxin a mold produces varies depending on what it is competing with—other molds, bacteria, insects that feed on it, and so forth. It's as if mold has a medicine cabinet of antibiotics to choose from.

Some people assume that if you test a home and don't find spores in the air, there is no health concern. This is an incorrect conclusion. If things have been wet, and mold started to grow, there will be mycelium and chemical residuals from the mold's metabolism that are known to affect the health of those occupying a building.

In the next stage of growth, mold produces spores to reproduce. Mold spores are like pollen spores, waiting in the wind to blow away. If a leak is fixed and the materials dry out, mold will stop growing. Some believe dry mold is dead. A gardener knows it as over-wintering. Mold goes dormant, waiting to get wet again. The dry spores remain intact and are dispersed when disturbed by air currents or vibrations. Dry (dormant) mold can be a hazard in terms of the number of spores dispersed.

What Can It Do to Me?

All molds are allergenic and potentially toxigenic. Response depends on a person's immune system, dose, and the duration of exposure. Chronic exposure may lead to allergies or asthma in otherwise healthy people. Dead (non-viable is the correct term) spores are still a concern.

What Your Builder Should Know

Allergens and toxins are not neutralized with bleach and chemicals. For mold remediation to be effective, mold must be removed. Symptoms of exposure to mold and moisture include:

- allergies

- cold and flu symptoms

- burning eyes and itchy skin

- difficulty breathing

- dry, hacking cough, sore throat

- headache

- nosebleeds

- fatigue

Preventing Mold

To prevent mold requires preventing leaks and moisture intrusion. The top three places leaks occur are around windows and doors, places the weather barrier fails (housewrap) on the outside walls, and around showers. Water leaks inside exterior walls if the openings around windows are not flashed properly before the windows are inserted. Plastic housewrap used to make houses air-tight is not as waterproof as what can be made using two layers of traditional, Grade D building paper.

Mold

Shower bladders, liners that wrap around showers behind the tile, are often installed incorrectly and leak. For
additional information, please read *Mold Money: How to
Save Thousands of Dollars on Mold Remediation and Make
Sure the Mold is Gone.*

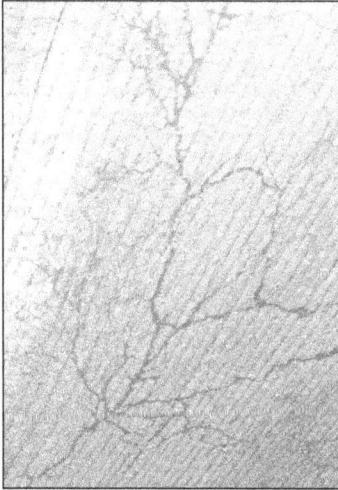

**Mycelium (mold roots),
spidering on wet wood
under a floor.**

What Your Builder Should Know

Electromagnetic Fields (EMFs)

What Is It?

When the power to a house is turned on, the wiring is energized, creating electric fields. The wires are at 120 volts (V). The plastic jacket that protects wires does not prevent electric fields from extending into the living space. The electric fields drop with distance from the wires. The issue is it's hard to get away from wires, and anything plugged emits an electric field, even if it is turned off. The voltage induced on a body can be measured using a multimeter, the same meter an electrician uses to measure voltage on wires. The voltage on the body of someone occupying a home is typically between 1 and 3 V.

When something is turned on, current flows, and an additional type of field is created—a magnetic field. The strength of the magnetic field will depend on how much current is flowing and if the house is wired properly.

What Your Builder Should Know

Dirty electricity (DE) is a type of EMF created by devices that require low power, less than 120V. A transformer in the circuits of these devices lowers the power. DE is a product of the transformation. These devices include energy saving light bulbs, dimmer switches, chargers for cell phones, computers, and appliances that contain digital clocks or LCD displays (almost all modern appliances).

What Can It Do to Me?

A 1995 booklet by the National Institute of Environmental Health Services (NIEHS) and U.S. Department of Energy lists the potential health effects from exposure to EMFs. These include a decrease in the hormone melatonin, alterations in the immune system, changes in biorhythms, changes in brain activity, and changes in heart rate[1]. A study funded by Kaiser Permanente found the risk of miscarriage increased for women exposed to magnetic fields above 2.5 milligauss (mG)[2]. Wireless transmission is listed as a possible carcinogen by the International Agency for Research on Cancer.

Minimizing EMFs

We can't get live without electricity, but there are things we can do to minimize the fields. Wiring errors are a significant reason for an increase in magnetic fields. This book provides recommendations for building a house to minimize wiring errors. Electric fields can nearly be eliminated using the types of wiring that will be suggested.

It is not practical to shield a house from radio frequencies (cellular antennas). Although it is possible, an engineer is required to design the material specifications, and the shielding materials are expensive.

It's important to not build a house where the ambient fields from power lines are high. Magnetic fields from power lines cannot be shielded. For additional information about EMFs, please read *Unplugged—How to Find and Get Rid of EMFs in Your Home.*

....

(1) *Questions and Answers About EMF, Electric and Magnetic Fields Associated with the Use of Electric Power.* National Institute of Environmental Health Services and U.S. Department of Energy. U.S. Government Printing Office. Washington, D.C. January, 1995.

(2) "Exposure to Magnetic Field Non-Ionizing Radiation and the Risk of Miscarriage: A Prospective Cohort Study." De-Kun Li, Hong Chen, Jeannette R. Ferber, Roxana Odouli & Charles Quesenberry. 2017.

What Your Builder Should Know

Volatile Organic Compounds (VOCs)

A chemical is considered a volatile organic compound (VOC) if it readily off-gases at room temperature. Every material off-gases, including products labeled zero-VOC. The term zero-VOC is based on testing a material for a limited set of compounds and the amount of off-gassing from them being below a limit set by the standard used to test them. Standards vary as to what is considered acceptable. The top contributors responsible for high levels of VOCs in a home are paint, carpet, kitchen cabinets, and particleboard.

There are sixty million known compounds[1]. When the air in a home is tested, the laboratory results are pages long. There are compounds the lab cannot identify, compounds formed when compounds react with each other. An educated guess of the identity of a compound is made based on the weight of the molecule, number of carbon atoms it contains, and how atoms are chained together. It's often unknown how a compound may affect the occupants.

What Your Builder Should Know

Just because there isn't a smell doesn't mean there are no chemicals in the air. Homeowners get used to the way a house smells or may ignore a smell. Some chemicals are odorless. Polyurethane in rigid and spray foams is an example. Although a manufacturer may say there is no off-gassing, there is off-gassing of toluene and di-isocyantes. There is no hint they are present except for symptoms—eye, nose, and respiratory irritation. Another example is formaldehyde. Between 10% and 20% of people are susceptible to formaldehyde at concentrations below its odor threshold. The chemicals commonly detected in homes include:

Benzene	Ethanol
Toluene	Hexanal
Methylene chloride	Pinene
Ethylbenzene	Camphene
Xylene	Terpinene
Styrene	Limonene
Dichlorobenzene	Nonanal
Naphthalene	Propylbenzene
Propylene	Acetaldehyde
Chloro-1,1-difluoroethane	Trimethylbenzene
Isopropanol	Isopropyltoluene
Acetone	Propanol

Volatile Organic Compounds

What Can It Do to Me?

The #1 symptom when there is a high level of VOCs in a home is eye, nose, and throat irritation. Studies show this is also the top symptom that a building needs additional ventilation. Some VOCs produce irritating odors; some are toxic; some carcinogenic. Other symptoms associated with VOCs include:

- Immune effects
- Hypersensitivity
- Allergies
- Asthma
- Cellular effects such as cancer
- Difficulty concentrating
- Tiredness
- Fatigue
- Headache
- Nausea
- Hoarseness

Natural gas and propane are significant VOC pollutants. Small amounts compromise the immune system and can increase asthma, cause waking with shortness of breath, and tingling sensations in the extremities.

Semi-VOCs

Chemicals that don't off-gas readily at room temperature are called semi-volatile organic compounds (SVOCs). The pathway for exposure is dust. Chemicals attach to dust particles. Children and pets are more susceptible because of their low body weight, activities, and contact with the floor. Sources of SVOCs include:

- flame retardants
- pesticides (including water-based permethrins)
- phthalates (softeners added to plastics and PVC)
- treated carpet
- biocides
- treated wood

Do not buy a house with a built-in pest control system. The use of pest control one year before birth to three years after is associated with an increased risk of childhood leukemia[2].

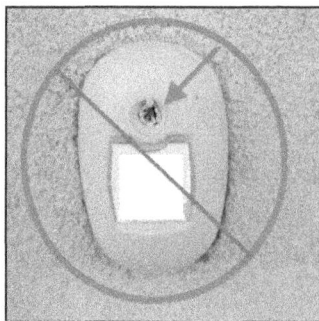

Clearing the Air

Green builders like to say, "Build it tight. Ventilate it right." They build a house airtight and are good at it. They do a poor job of ventilating them. I suggest a new slogan—"Build it right, ventilate it with all of your might." There's no such thing as too much ventilation. Do the best building a house with healthy materials and ventilate it as best you can.

Volatile Organic Compounds

(1) www.cas.org/support/documentation/chemical-substances. The CAS REGISTRY[sm] of chemical substance information contains more than 154 million unique chemical substances and 68 million sequences.

(2) "Critical Windows of Exposure to Household Pesticides and Risk of Childhood Leukemia." *Environmental Health Perspectives*, 2002 Sep; 110(9): 955–960.

What Your Builder Should Know

Dust

The common particles in dust from construction include: drywall (gypsum), sawdust (an allergen), concrete, silica (a carcinogen), fiberglass, cellulose, carpet fibers, and dust from cutting plastic and PVC pipe—cadmium, zinc, and tin.

When investigating a house in which people complain about being sick, there are two common tests that are performed. The first is to test for mold. If mold is not

Sample #:	1		Description:	House Dust	
Nuisance Particulate:		(%)	**Biological Particulate:**		(%)
Asbestos:	(Total)	ND	Mold:	(Total)	2
	Fibrous Glass	2	Pollen:	(Total)	ND
	Mineral Wool	ND	Diatoms:	(Total)	<1
	Ceramic Fibers	ND	Insect Fragments:	(Total)	ND
Glass:	Fragments	ND			
Common Particulate:		(%)			(%)
Cellulosic:	Processed	15		Iron Oxides	5
	Natural	ND		Aluminum Oxide	ND
	Wood	3		Zinc Oxide	ND
	Paper Dust	25		Paint Dust	<1
	Starch	5		Quartz	5
Synthetic:	(Total)	2		Calcite/ Dolomite	10
				Gypsum/ Anhydrite	5
				Clay	7
	Human Hair	1		Cement	ND
	Animal Hair	ND		Mica	3
	Skin Fragments	ND		Halite	1

Laboratory results for a sample of house dust.

present, the next test is for chemicals (VOCs). If the laboratory results do not show harmful or unusual chemicals in the air, the final test is an analysis of the house dust. The laboratory will use various methods to identify the particles in the dust. It can be a challenge determining which particles are responsible for irritation or illness. It's difficult to say what level of a particle is too much. Small levels are known to cause allergies and irritation.

What Can It Do to Me?

The components in dust trigger allergies and can cause one to feel something is not right and healthy in a new home. It's simpler to keep the construction site clean, clean as workers go, and prevent an accumulation of dust. If you have allergies after you move in, you may wonder what the culprit is and have a difficult time figuring it out.

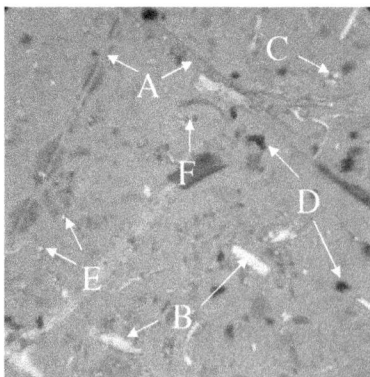

Figure 1: PLM image of the sample
A: Fibrous glass
B: Cellulose
C: Starch
D: Clay
E: Quartz
F: Gypsum

Water

Water is a complex topic. The possible contaminants and methods of filtration are numerous. City water is straightforward. The usually contaminants are chlorine and fluoride. The typical treatment is a whole-house tank system with carbon to remove chlorine, and a reverse-osmosis (RO) filter in the kitchen for drinking water. An RO filter removes 98% of most contaminants.

The quality of well water varies from pristine to undrinkable. A water testing report is required to determine what types of filters are required.

Chlorine

Chlorine reacts with organic matter to form by-products called trihalomethanes (THMs). The Environmental Protection Agency (EPA) limits the amount of THMs allowed in water. When the limit is reached, a city cannot add additional chlorine. The City of Los Angeles, for example, installed an ozone water treatment plant to supplement its use of chlorine.

Fluoride

The type of fluoride added to drinking water (sodium fluoride) is different than what should be used by a healthy dentist (calcium fluoride). Fluoride added to drinking water is obtained by salvaging waste by-products from various industries. Fluoridation is associated with aluminum, another by-product. Neither aluminum nor fluoride is removed with a carbon filter. An RO filter is required.

Bacteria

Homeowners on a well test for fecal coliform bacteria, the type associated with being too close to the septic field and sewage.

Hard Water

Hard water is composed of calcium and magnesium carbonates, minerals that clog pipes and cause white spots on glasses coming out of the dishwasher. The minerals are a nuisance, not a health hazard. A water softener is required to treat hard water.

Radon

Radon causes lung cancer. If high levels are present, there may be exposure when showering or running the dishwasher. With an airtight house this is a concern. A whole-house carbon tank water system removes radon.

Bromine

Bromine is as toxic as chlorine. A healthier sanitizer to treat a pool or tub uses copper and silver ions. Copper prevents algae; silver kills bacteria.

Lead

Lead causes brain damage and learning disabilities in children; in men, hypertension and heart attack; in women, fertility problems. There is no safe level. Corrosion of old plumbing is the primary source. The city report does not account for lead in the pipes in an older home. Almost all water filters remove lead. New homes should have lead-free pipes and solder.

Copper, plastic, and PVC (vinyl chloride)

Depending on what kind of water pipes you have, there may be plastic or copper introduced into the water. Stainless steel pipes are required for pure drinking water. Most filters remove copper. An RO removes plastic.

Arsenic

Liver, kidney, and bladder cancers are associated with arsenic. High levels require a specialized media in a tank system.

Uranium

The city report may be unreliable. A special test is required for the accurate measurement of the level of uranium in water. To filter uranium requires a media in a tank system. An RO filter removes uranium. The issue is that an RO filter removes 98%, but 2% may be too much.

Nitrates

Nitrates may be abundant in areas with a history of farming or livestock. Run-off from fertilizer is a source. This can be an issue for those on a well. Nitrates are hazardous to infants. A bacterium in an infant's stomach converts it to a compound that reduces the oxygen capacity of the blood. Blue Baby Syndrome and spontaneous abortions are associated. Test the water.

Iron

Too much iron is more a nuisance than a health hazard. A softener can remove it if the level is low. If the water is brown to orange, a tank type system is required.

Step by Step

Choosing a Lot

What It Is

These are things to consider before purchasing a lot or picking one available from a builder.

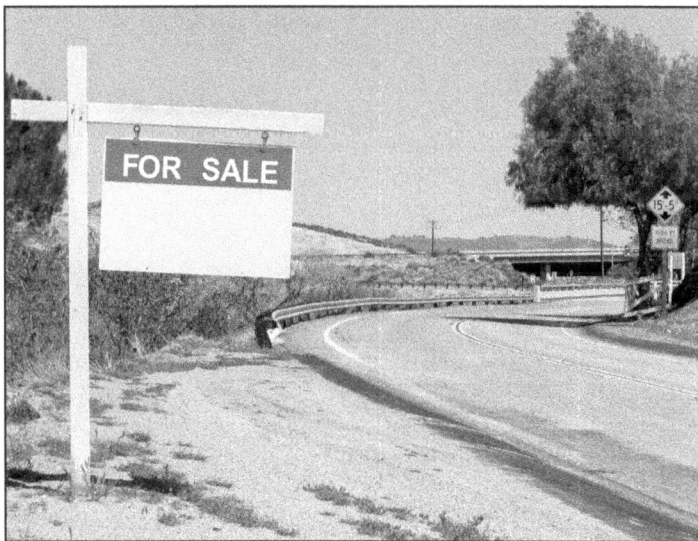

What Your Builder Should Know

Categories of Concern

Noise
Pollution
Traffic
Mold
EMFs

Shortcuts and Standard Practices

A builder doesn't like you watching. The bigger the home-building company, the more likely you may be told to stay away except for a few walk-through inspections. There are commonly two walk-through inspections. The first is after the house is framed; the other is when the house is finished. A homeowner is normally not allowed on-site in between.

What Can Go Wrong Here

The lot may be too close to power lines. There may be high magnetic fields from underground power lines.

The land might slope towards the spot you intend to build, causing water to collect next to the house. An extensive drainage system may be required to prevent mold. To work, drain pipes need to drain to daylight. If a lot is flat or a neighbor's house is next to yours, there may be nowhere for water to go.

Choosing a Lot

You may have visited the lot on a weekend or in the evening. Other times there might be noise and traffic.

Pesticides are sprayed near railroad tracks and highways for weed and fire prevention.

There may have been illegal dumping.

Recommendations

Visit the site on a weekend and on a weekday. Visit in the morning and late afternoon.

Investigate nearby businesses. Find out the potential for noise, traffic, and pollution. You don't want an auto-body shop or dry cleaners behind the fence in your backyard.

Walk the land. Keep an eye out for mounds of dirt from illegal dumping, cleared areas, and odors. Commercial investors request a Phase I Environmental Assessment. This shows locations of underground storage tanks from gas stations, historical aerial photos, and ground water data. Contact Environmental Data Resources at (800) 352-0050, edrnet.com.

Measure the level of electromagnetic fields (EMFs). The term electromagnetic fields is a catch-all and includes electric, magnetic, and high-frequency fields. We are concerned about magnetic fields from power lines. Buy or borrow a gauss meter. Walk the four corners of the property. Walk the area where the house and yard will be. Note any reading above zero. If readings are above 0.5 mG, contact an EMF consultant to make sure you took accurate readings.

Magnetic fields from underground power lines can be as large as those from above ground. Avoid buying a house where power lines run under the sidewalk on your side of the street unless you have measured near the sidewalk and found the readings acceptable.

It is expensive to rent a meter to accurately measure EMFs from cell towers. Do your best looking for cell towers. Radiation goes through glass easier than walls. If the house is on a hill or has views of the city, consider shielding the windows. Additional information on shielding can be found in *Unplugged: How to Find and Get Rid of EMFs in Your Home.*

Give This to Your Builder

The owner has the right to come on-site and check on progress each day as long as it does not interfere with work or safety.

Permits

(Consider this step if there will be a pool or well)

What It Is

Permits are obtained from the city and electric company.

Categories of Concern

EMFs

Shortcuts and Standard Practices

Normally there is one main electric panel and one service connection from the electric company to the house. Power to a pool or a well is normally supplied from the main house using a sub-panel. The issue is that the current from panels can flow back to the electric company through the ground instead of the wires. This may cause EMFs in the house.

The issue can be avoided by supplying a pool and a well each with their own main electric panels, connected directly to the transformer the electric company uses to supply power. That way, any current flowing though the ground at the pool site or in the well does not affect the house. To have more than one main panel requires a special permit. It's like having more than one service hookup.

What Can Go Wrong Here

If you change your mind and decide you want the pool and well to have their own main electric panels, you will need to get a revised permit and wait to start building.

Recommendations

Tell the general contractor to tell the electrician that you need a permit to have service entry electrical panels for each a pool and a well. Do this when you first meet with the builder.

Give This to Your Builder

Obtain a permit for electrical power to power a pool with its own main panel connected directly to the transformer.

Obtain a permit for electrical power to power a well with its own main panel connected directly to the transformer.

These should not be sub-panels from the house.

Creating a List of Approved Materials

What It Is

There is a section in construction specifications, General Requirements, that lists acceptable and non-acceptable products.

What Can Go Wrong Here

The builder has to start ordering materials. It's unreasonable to object to a material without stating your requirements before construction begins.

The Alternatives

Most green labels are based on environmental concerns, not air quality. There are only two labeling organizations that test the air with their products applied to samples: Indoor Advantage and GREENGUARD. GREENGUARD Gold has the strictest requirements.

What Your Builder Should Know

Allowable emissions	GREENGUARD (The same LEED® requires if the air is tested)	GREENGUARD Gold
Total VOC	500 ug/m2	220 ug/m2
Formaldehyde	50 ppb	7.3 ppb

Suggestions for Researching Products

• Check if a product meets the requirements for the State of California Collaborative for High Performance Schools (CHPS). The database is on-line.

• Avoid products with "inert" or "other" ingredients.

• Download the Safety Data Sheet (SDS) or Material Safety Data Sheet (MSDS).

• The Household Products Database of the National Institutes of Health is a good resource.

• Look for the Safer Choice label. To obtain it, a manufacturer is required to disclose all the ingredients to the EPA. If a formula is a trade secret, the EPA keeps the ingredients confidential after reviewing them.

Specify how a substitute will be chosen if a material is not available.

Approved Materials

Recommendations

Copy and paste the references in the Appendix into the specifications you give the builder.

Specify an individual, foreman, or supervisor whose job it is to ensure the specifications are followed and prevent unapproved materials from being delivered and used.

Give This to Your Builder

01 25 13 PRODUCT SUBSTITUTION PROCEDURES

No product may be substituted unless agreed upon in writing by the owner or architect.

The procedure for product substitution is:

1 The contractor should submit a request to the owner or architect. The request should be accompanied by complete product data, including a list of ingredients and safety data sheets.

2 The contractor will obtain product samples and submit them with the request.

3 The request shall note any changes using the product may cause to construction, a narrative comparing the substitute to the original product, the estimated cost of using the substitute, and if a work order change is required.

01 31 00 PROJECT MANAGEMENT COORDINATION

Specify an individual, foreman, or supervisor whose job it is to ensure the specifications are followed and to prevent unapproved materials from being accepted for delivery.

What Your Builder Should Know

01 42 00 REFERENCES

This section shall contain drawings, references, standards, and codes. Copy and include the references in the Appendix.

01 61 00 COMMON PRODUCT REQUIREMENTS

The owner will list prohibited products.

The builder will specify products that have code requirements.

01 64 00 OWNER-FURNISHED PRODUCTS

List products the owner will provide and deliver.

Post a Sign

Give This to Your Builder

01 58 13 TEMPORARY PROJECT SIGNAGE

A sign shall be posted that says the following:

This house is being constructed as a healthy house.

Only specified materials, products, and procedures may be used. A copy of the specifications, approved materials, and construction techniques are available from the foreman. Substitutes must be approved in writing.

Smoking in or near the building and the garage is prohibited.

The use of pesticides and antimicrobials is prohibited.

Gas-powered machines, gas generators, and gas heaters are not allowed inside the house or garage.

Spills of fuel, solvents, or chemicals must be avoided. If a spill occurs, report it immediately and clean it up using the approved cleaning products.

Heaters may not be used to accelerate drying plaster, paint, tile, or finishes. Fans and dehumidifiers may be used, placing fans at forty-five degree angles to walls to wick moisture.

What Your Builder Should Know

A Well Is Drilled

What It Is

If required, a well is drilled.

Categories of Concern

Water quality

What Can Go Wrong Here

The flow rate may be too low or the water too contaminated to treat. You may have to truck water in or install a complex filtration system.

Recommendations

Have the water tested before construction begins. A cost-effective test that checks for ninety-four contaminants may be ordered from National Testing Laboratories. Collect and send a sample to radon.com to be tested for radon. Collect a sample and hand-deliver it to a local laboratory to be tested for fecal coliform bacteria.

Install an ultraviolet light (UV) system on the line coming from the well.

If the water testing report is good, the only additional filter you may need is in the kitchen for drinking. A good supplier for water filters is Krudico (800) 211-1369. You need to take care of this yourself, and tell your builder what kind of filters you want and where to put them.

Give This to Your Builder

02 24 13.43 WATER ASSESSMENT

Water should be tested before construction begins.

33 11 13 POTABLE WATER SUPPLY WELLS

The well casing shall extend above the ground to prevent the well from being contaminated with run-off.

The Foundation Is Staked

What It Is

Decide where the house will be on the lot and its orientation.

Categories of Concern

Noise
Traffic
Mold
EMFs

What Can Go Wrong Here

The site may be graded in a manner that the concrete slab is level with the land. This is called "at grade" and is not high enough. The finished slab must be four inches above the ground.

The service entry for electrical power may be on the same side of the house as the bedrooms.

Wires may need to go over bedrooms to reach other parts of the house.

The regulators on gas meters leak to relieve pressure. You don't want a gas meter near a bedroom window or the fresh-air intake for the ventilation system.

The Alternatives

When designing the blueprints, consider the locations of the bedrooms relative to the electric panel and gas meter (if there is gas or propane). Try to place the bedrooms at the opposite side of the house from where the utilities enter.

Position the house as far as possible from the road.

Avoid building next to a hill and in locations water could collect next to the house.

Rough Grading and Excavating

What It Is

Trees, rocks, and dirt are moved to create the yard, drive-way, and drainage. Trenches are dug for the foundation. If the house will not be connected to a sewer, a septic tank and drain field are put in.

Categories of Concern

Mold

Shortcuts and Standard Practices

The builder may do the least amount of work required to level the land. He or she may be in hurry to pour the foundation. Consideration may not be given to site drainage and keeping water away from the house.

What Can Go Wrong Here

As the house is being built, it may appear that there is a few inches of clearance between the top of the slab and ground. After the house is built and the landscaping is finished, dirt is pushed up next to the house.

Check for This

Look for a sign posted stating this is a healthy home. If there is a swimming pool or a well, look for the second and third electric panels. The panels should connect directly to the transformer, not the main electric panel in the house.

Give This to Your Builder

31 10 00 SITE CLEARING

The owner will specify requirements for protecting plants, tress, grass, and rocks.

31 22 00 GRADING

Water should drain away from the house, around the perimeter, with a minimum grade of 5%.

31 23 00 EXCAVATION AND FILL

Back-fill and compact the soil to raise the level of the finished slab so that it is a minimum of four inches above the ground when the house is finished and the landscaping is added.

Temporary Utilities

What It Is

Power, water, and a portable toilet are required during construction.

Categories of Concern

Mold

Shortcuts and Standard Practices

It's standard for contractors to bring gas-powered tools into the house and garage. In the winter, gas-powered space heaters may be used.

Some workers take pride in their work; others leave a mess as if they are college freshmen in a dormitory. They don't clean up (sawdust, scraps of lumber, drywall, and so forth) and leave soda bottles and trash from lunch lying around.

What Can Go Wrong Here

The main product of gas combustion is water vapor. If gas-powered generators are used inside, depending on how cold it is outside, condensation and mold can result. Mold will grow inside walls where it is not visible.

Do You Know?

I received a call from a builder who asked if I knew about condensation. His question seemed odd, as he wanted an inspection of mold that he believed was due to a roof leak. The house was under construction. The inside of every exterior wall was covered with mold. The mold was obvious. The source of moisture was not. The builder wanted to blame it on the roofer. I did not find a roof leak that explained that much mold.

I went back to my office to write a report and wrestled to make a conclusion in regard to the source of the moisture. I took a break and went to dinner. One the way back I stopped at the house. In the middle of the living room was a portable 3-burner camp stove. The burners were on full in attempts to heat the house. Along each exterior wall, pointing at the walls, were propane heaters. The builder was trying to dry the plaster. It was winter. The main product of combustion is water vapor. The heaters were driving moisture into the walls. The outside temperature was below dew point, the warmest a surface may be before condensation (dripping water) occurs. As the vapor reached the outside wall, it condensed and soaked the walls. This explained why every exterior wall had mold, not just one with a roof leak.

Recommendations

Do not allow the contractor or subcontractors to use gas-powered generators inside the house or garage.

Give This to Your Builder

01 51 00 Temporary Utilities

Gas generators and gas heaters are prohibited in the house and garage. Using electric heaters powered by a gas generator outside, away from the house, is acceptable.

Heaters should not be used to accelerate drying plaster, paint, or texture. If needed, fans and dehumidifiers may be used, placing the fans at forty-five degree angles to the walls to wick moisture off of them.

Temporary Sanitary Facilities

Use of the bathrooms and toilets inside the house is prohibited. The builder shall provide and maintain portable chemical toilets for workers.

Temporary Closures

Provide temporary weatherproofing of exterior walls, roofs, and penetrations for doors and windows as needed to keep materials and the structure dry.

What Your Builder Should Know

TEMPORARY FLOOR PROTECTION

Cover flooring as it is installed to protect it from damage and construction traffic.

PROTECTION OF INSTALLED WORK

Protect installed finish carpentry, cabinets, floors, and surfaces from soil, wear and tear. Use craft paper and temporary mats as necessary. Cover cabinets as they are installed with polyethylene plastic and temporary tape to keep dust out of them.

PARKING

Designate a location for temporary parking. Restrict parking as needed to protect native landscaping, soil, bushes, and trees.

WASTE MANAGEMENT

The site shall be kept clean and in orderly condition.

Maintain a waste container with a lid.

SMOKING

Smoking on the premise is prohibited, including outside and in the garage.

Underground Plumbing and Electrical

What It Is

Plumbing pipes and electrical conduit are put in the ground before the foundation and slab are poured. This is called rough-in plumbing.

Categories of Concern

Water quality
EMFs
Radon

Shortcuts and Standard Practices

You asked for a radon mitigation system, and the builder said there is one. What they meant is pipes are installed under the slab. They may not install the fans. They may be waiting for the house to be tested after it is built.

It's standard to cut, glue, and install pipe inside. If glue spills on concrete and dust from plastic being sawed collects, workers assume it will be covered by paint and flooring.

What Can Go Wrong Here

You didn't think about what kind of water pipes you want. There are two issues: EMFs and water quality. Metal water pipes are supposed to be grounded to the main electric panel. This electrifies the slab with small voltages. Using cross-linked polyethylene (PEX) or PVC negates the issue, as these are non-conductive.

The Alternatives

Decide on what type of water pipes you want. The options are: PEX, copper, stainless steel, and PVC. PEX has been known to leak. Some types of PEX are thought to be more prone to failure, and it's thought the issue has been resolved. If your builder is used to using PEX, it makes it easier to minimize EMFs. EMFs occur when metal pipes touch concrete. PEX, like plastic, does not conduct.

PVC is cheap and commonly used. PVC manufactured in China has lead. Stainless steel is expensive but offers unmatched purity of drinking water and lack of corrosion. Copper is common. Copper pipes leach copper into drinking water. There are issues with corrosion and pin-

Plumbing and Electrical

hole leaks. Installing dielectric unions minimizes the risk of corrosion. Most water filters remove lead and copper.

To minimize electric fields, use metal clad wire instead of the normal plastic-jacketed romex.

Recommendations

Specify health care facility (HCF) or electrical metallic tubing (EMT) as the type of wiring. This prevents 98% of the electric fields that result from house wiring.

Tell the builder you want a radon mitigation system and to include the fans. There should be a switch to turn the fans off if test results indicate the level of radon is low after the house is built.

Give This to Your Builder

22 11 16 DOMESTIC WATER PIPING

A dielectric union should be inserted between different types of metal pipe to reduce the potential for corrosion, pitting, and pinhole leaks.

If the water pipes are metal, prevent them from touching the concrete. The issue is EMFs. Metal pipes are bonded to the ground at the main electric panel. A solution is to run metal pipes through PVC where pipes penetrate the slab.

Prior to occupancy, run the water to flush the pipes of flux, soldering, glue, and residual particles.

What Your Builder Should Know

26 05 33 13 CONDUIT FOR ELECTRICAL SYSTEMS

Wiring material shall be Health Care Facility (HCF) or Electrical Metallic Tubing (EMT). The outer metal casing must serve as an equipment grounding conductor. Electrical boxes and bushings connected to electrical boxes shall be metal. 240V cables have two 120V hot conductors of opposite polarity, thus creating the cancellation of electric fields without the need for special cable.

31 21 13 RADON MITIGATION

Install a radon mitigation system under the slab. Consult with a local radon mitigation contractor for specifications. A fan shall be installed. Label the switch and the circuit breaker that controls the fan.

Do not put the fan for a radon mitigation system outside near a bedroom window.

After construction is complete, a short-term radon test should be performed with the mitigation system off. If the results exceed the EPA limit of 4.0 piC/l, the fan should be turned on and a second short-term test performed.

Footing and Foundation

What It Is

The foundation is poured into wooden forms and trenches.

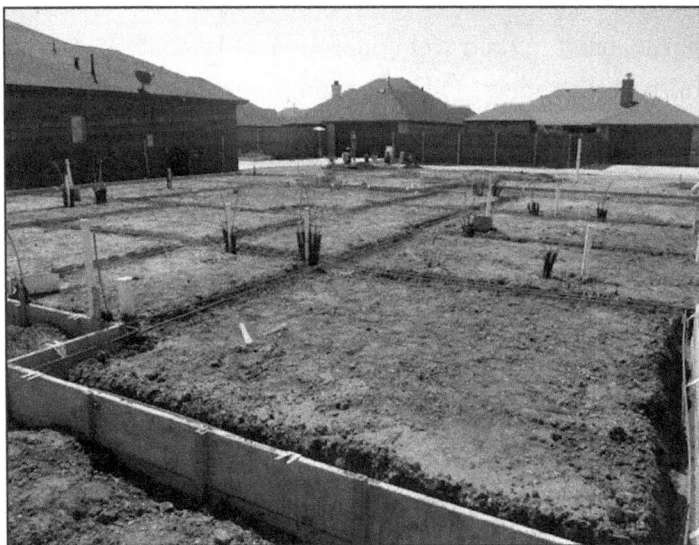

Categories of Concern

Pesticides
Mold

Shortcuts and Standard Practices

It's common to treat soil for termites.

What Can Go Wrong Here

The builder may treat the soil with pesticides without asking if it is required.

Forms used to hold wet concrete may be coated with an oil-based product. Oil that remains on concrete causes odors in the home.

The Alternatives

Do not have a basement or a crawlspace. Build on a concrete slab. A lot of air quality and health problems are due to basements and crawlspaces. If you must have a crawlspace, build it as mini-basement and heat and cool it as a normal room in the house. Pour a concrete slab in the crawlspace. For suggestions on how to build a crawlspace or a basement, see *Builder's Guide* by Joseph Lstiburek. The details depend on your climate and type of construction.

Footing and Foundation

Do not treat for termites unless they are known to be a problem in your location. The effective treatment depends on the type of termite. Keeping things dry helps prevent termites regardless of where you live. A promising suggestion is the installation of a fine-woven stainless steel mesh barrier cloth called Termimesh™. It is placed under and around the foundation to prevent subterranean termites.

Before the slab is poured, tape Termimesh™ around plumbing pipes and electrical conduits to prevent termites entering through gaps between the poured concrete and pipes.

Desiccating dusts such as diatomaceous earth and silica aerogel may be used to prevent dry wood termites. It dries out a termite's shell. Swimming pool grade is ineffective. Use food grade, without a pyrethrin.

Give This to Your Builder

03 11 00 CONCRETE FORMING

Petroleum-based form oils are prohibited. The following are acceptable:

- vegetable oil
- an acceptable paint
- BioForm™ (water-based)
- Crete-Lease® (soy-based)
- DUOGARD® (water-based)

What Your Builder Should Know

07 11 00 DAMP PROOFING

Damp proofing should be applied to walls in contact with soil or below grade. Use an acceptable product. Before applying the coating, fill voids, cracks, and holes in the walls with cement mortar and allow the mortar to dry. Care should be taken during back-filling and subsequent construction activities to prevent damaging damp-proofed surfaces.

The damp-proof coatings may be an asphalt type product or a self-adhering (peel and stick) membrane.

Asphalt Products

Asphalt cannot grow mold. Anything that comes in contact with it is protected. It's how they used to build ships. Consider the two-coat system of Henry #910 Asphalt Primer and Henry® 793 Premium Foundation Coating, Trowel Grade. This is a solvent-based product and has an odor when applied. Take care to avoid drips and spills on surfaces that will not be covered by the back-filling of dirt. Do not apply when it could rain within 24 hours. The wall should be dry before applying. Wire-brush and use a broom to clear loose dirt and residual mortar from the walls. Apply the prime coat and allow it to dry. Using a trowel (and putty knife as needed), apply a coat of Henry® 793 Foundation Coating, Trowel Grade a minimum of 1/8-inch thick. The coating should be applied in a continuous film, filling and spreading around joints and grooves and penetrating into crevices and corners. Carry the coating up to finished grade. Allow the coating to set two days before back-filling.

Membrane Products

Membranes can be more effective at preventing water intrusion than tar. Make sure to follow the manufacturer's instructions, overlap layers, and use a roller to press it on.

MEL-ROL® by W.R. Meadows is a rolled, self-adhering waterproofing membrane, 56 mil thick.

Footing and Foundation

31 31 00 SOIL TREATMENT

Do not treat for termites unless approved by the owner.

33 41 43 SYNTHETIC-MEDIA FRENCH DRAINS

Where a wall is below grade, a French drain should be installed
after applying the waterproof coating. Start by installing a heavy-
duty polypropylene drainage fabric at the bottom of the stem wall
(trench). The fabric allows water to pass but not dirt. This is a
liner into which the pipes and gravel are placed. Use a fabric 4 feet
wide. The trench should be 2 feet wide. The fabric should cover
the bottom plus one foot on each side, to be lapped over the pipe
and gravel before back-filling.

Pour a 2-inch bed of 3/4-inch gravel into the bottom of the trench,
onto the fabric. The gravel should not have small particles that
can clog pipes. Install a 4-inch diameter flexible, corrugated
HDPE-pipe drainpipe on top of the gravel. Use a contiguous
section or the proper fittings if required to create a longer section
to drain the pipe to daylight. Do not use a pipe pre-wrapped in
filter fabric (a sock). Do not wrap pipe with fabric. The fabric
should wrap around the stone and the pipe.

Install pipes with the holes facing down so that water can rise into
them. It's acceptable to have perforations on more than one side.
At least one side with perforations should face down. The pipes
should slope away from the house, downward, a minimum of 1 to
1.5 feet along the wall. Verify that water collects in the pipes and
drains to daylight using a hose to fill the pipes with water before
continuing.

Pour 3-4 inches of 3/4-inch gravel on top of the pipes. Wrap the
drainage cloth fabric over the top of the pipes and gravel before
back-filling with soil.

What Your Builder Should Know

Slab

What It Is

After the building inspector inspects the foundation, the slab is poured.

Categories of Concern

Mold
Oil odors
EMFs
VOCs

Shortcuts and Standard Practices

A vapor barrier is usually not installed, or it is installed poorly. The builder may use poly sheeting from the garden department. The builder may worry that the vapor barrier will be damaged when the concrete is being poured and use sand as a couchin. Sand holds moisture. The vapor barrier may not be lapped over the footer or inspected for tears. Penetrations around plumbing and electrical pipes are usually not sealed.

It's common to put rebar in concrete even though it is not required.

It's common to add water to concrete as it's being poured to make it easier to work with. A builder may not understand that adding water makes concrete weaker and increases its vapor permeability.

It's not common to cover a slab after the concrete is poured to cure it.

It's not common after a slab is dry to inspect it for cracks and use silicon caulk to seal cracks and around penetrations at pipes. I had a client who had to get permission to go on-site and do it himself.

What Can Go Wrong Here

If a vapor barrier is not installed correctly, moisture evaporates into the house. This can cause mold to grow under carpet and in places with less ventilation, such as closets. If the vapor barrier was not sealed around penetrations in the slab at plumbing pipes and electrical conduits, mold odors, radon, and pests can get inside.

Rigid foam may have been installed under the slab or between the foundation and the slab. Rigid foam off-gases freon (HCF-142B) and is detected in the air in homes.

Slab

Concrete becomes weaker and more vapor-permeable as water is added.

Rebar distributes electromagnetic fields. There may be a constant, low voltage on bare feet in contact with a concrete slab. This is because the electric code requires the electric panel to be grounded to metal water pipes and to rebar in the concrete.

The Alternatives

The options are to use rebar in the concrete slab or not. If reinforcement is required, use non-metallic fibers.

A vapor barrier is optional. Install one.

If the builder insists on using it, the best place to put rigid foam is on the exterior of the foundation. This insulates better than foam placed between the foundation and slab, and it prevents air quality and structural issues that occur when foam is placed under a slab or between the foundation and the slab.

Recommendations

Do not coat concrete forms with an oil-based product. Use a water-based product from the approved list.

Do not use rebar in the slab. If reinforcement is required, add non-metallic fibers to the concrete mix.

What Your Builder Should Know

Rebar in the footer (foundation) is OK.

Do not put rigid foam under the slab or between the slab and foundation. It's OK to put rigid foam on the exterior, the outermost part of the foundation.

Install a vapor barrier on the ground before the concrete is poured. Put the vapor barrier on top of a bed of coarse gravel. Seal the seams and penetrations around pipes with the sealant tape supplied by the manufacturer of the vapor barrier. Repair any tears with the tape.

Specify the details regarding the concrete water-to-cement ratio. The ratio should not exceed 0.45. Water should not be added to improve the workability of fresh concrete as it is poured.

Driveway Bridges

He used to build highway bridges. Then he moved to a small town and found a job at the community college as Chair of the construction department. He used the opportunity to teach the latest green building techniques. As students, we had a project to pour a driveway up a hill. We did not use rebar. He explained concrete wants to crack more where there is rebar—that's what control joints are for; you make concrete crack where you want it to, at the control joints, and seal the joints with silicon. Rebar, he said, is addictive. If you use it, you find you always need more.

Slab

Check for this when the builder says the slab is ready to be poured

Check that the pipes for radon mitigation are installed. Check that a vapor barrier is installed. The vapor barrier should be placed over a bed of gravel. Check that the seams on the vapor barrier and penetrations around pipes are sealed with the sealant tape supplied by the manufacturer of the vapor barrier. If rigid foam is used, make sure it's not under the slab and not between the slab and footer. It is permissible on the exterior side of the footer.

Check for this as concrete is being poured

As the concrete is delivered and poured, ensure water is not added to make it easier to work with. Ask for documentation and a sump test to ensure the water-to-cement ratio is no greater than 0.45.

After the pouring, make sure the slab is covered with burlap and cured for a week.

Check for this after the slab is poured, BEFORE framing begins

After the slab is dry, inspect it for cracks. Seal cracks with silicon caulk. Caulk around plumbing, electrical, and water pipes where they penetrate the slab.

What Your Builder Should Know

Check the clearance between the top of the slab and the ground. It needs to be at least four inches. Make sure water cannot collect next to the house. If water could collect next to the house, tell the builder to move dirt away from the slab and re-grade the landscape.

Give This to Your Builder

03 15 21 TERMITE, SOIL GAS, AND ODOR BARRIER

Before the slab is poured, after the vapor barrier is installed, use Termimesh™ or the sealant tape provided by the manufacturer of the vapor barrier to seal around pipe and conduit penetrations.

After the slab is dry, expansion joints and penetrations around plumbing, water pipes, and electrical conduits shall be sealed with 100% silicon caulk.

03 20 00 CONCRETE REINFORCING

Rebar is not permitted. If reinforcement is required, use fiberglass or polypropylene fibers, such as Fibermesh 650 or Novomesh 850/950. Ensure the concrete is mixed sufficiently after the fibers are added to the mix.

03 31 00 STRUCTURE CONCRETE

Use clean sand, gravel, and potable water. Water shall be free of color and odor. The supplier should provide a control sheet and document the weight and volume of the ingredients. Admixtures, accelerants, or retardants shall not be used. Comply with climatic parameters to obtain the desired strength and finish without additives. Air entrainment is acceptable for garage slabs.

Water should not be used on-site to improve the workability of concrete as it's being poured. If water needs to be added, measure the additional water and adjust the proportions of the ingredients in the mix to maintain a water-to-cement ratio of 0.45 or less. The water-to-cement ratio shall be no greater than 0.45. Individuals batching, mixing, and casting concrete should understand the importance of maintaining the specified water-to-cement ratio. Strength improves with lower water-to-cement ratios. Water permeability increases with higher ratios.

03 39 00 CONCRETE CURING

Concrete should be cured by ponding water on the surface and covering it with wet burlap three to seven days.

After the concrete is dry, silicon caulk shall be used to seal cracks, control joints, and penetrations around plumbing and electrical conduits.

07 26 16 BELOW-GRADE VAPOR RETARDERS

A 15-ml-thick polyethylene sheet shall cover the slab footprint prior to pouring the slab in compliance with *ASTM 1643-94, Standard Practice for Installation of Water Vapor Retarders Used in Contact with Earth or Granular Fill Under Concrete Slabs.*

Do not put sand on top of or under a vapor barrier. The vapor barrier should be put over a bed of six to eight inches of clean, dry, 1/2-inch coarse gravel (no fines or p-gravel). Roll the sheets out in the direction of the planned pouring. Overlap the seams six inches and seal the seams with the sealant tape supplied by the manufacturer of the vapor barrier material. Lap the vapor barrier over the footing and seal it to the foundation. Seal around electrical conduits and pipes penetrating the vapor barrier using the sealant tape. Inspect the vapor barrier before pouring. It needs to be watertight. Tears and punctures should be repaired.

Vapor barrier (retarder) products include:

- Perminator® 15 Mil. Order the sealant tape that goes with it. W.R. Meadows (800) 342-5976
- Stego® Wrap Vapor Barrier (15-Mil)

What Your Builder Should Know

Ventilation and HVAC

What It Is

The ventilator and HVAC (heating, ventilation, and air-conditioning) installations come later. They are presented here because HVAC subcontractors need to order parts. They need to know what type and how many ventilators will be installed, which rooms will have supply ducts, and where return ducts will be located.

Categories of Concern

Ventilation
Dust

Shortcuts and Standard Practices

Air conditioners are usually over-sized. The contractor doesn't want callbacks. (Contractors also make more money selling bigger systems.) The issue is dehumidification occurs only when the air-conditioning is running. If an air-conditioner is too big, it cools the house down and shuts off, stopping dehumidification. It will become muggy and uncomfortable. In humid climates mold can grow.

Unless required by code, a ventilator and ductwork for a ventilation system will not be installed. There are green builders who realize they should do something for ventilation. Somewhere they got the idea, and code considers it acceptable, they can use bathroom fans or the kitchen range hood for the ventilation system. If a builder says a house is "ventilated," this may be what is meant.

Air ducts leak. It's not standard to test air ducts to see where the leaks are and to repair them. The Residential Energy Services Network (RESNET) tester needs to be called to set up the blower door apparatus, and the HVAC contractor needs to be present to fix the leaks. The general contractor may have already scheduled the insulation company. Insulation will cover the ducts. The RESNET tester may not pour theatrical fog into the blower machine that is used to pressurize the ducts. Without fog, it's not possible to see where the leaks are. Without using fog, the RESNET tester will only say how leaky the ducts are, not where the leaks are.

Common practice is to say a furnace or air-conditioner has a high-efficiency particulate air (HEPA) filter. Few filters on the market are tested using a laser-particle counter, the accurate test. There are other tests manufacturers can use to claim a filter is a HEPA. Manufacturers make untrue claims regarding the effectiveness of ionizers, electronic air filters, electrostatic precipitators, and anti-bacterial and germicidal air cleaners. Most air filters are not effective at capturing small particles.

What Can Go Wrong Here

To satisfy any code requirements, the builder may reference ASHRAE (American Society of Heating, Refrigerating and Air-Conditioning Engineers) *Standard 62.2 Ventilation and Acceptable Indoor Air Quality in Low-Rise Residential Buildings*. Notice the title says *acceptable*, not *healthy*.

The builder or architect may hire an engineer to design blueprints for the ventilation system. The engineer will design the system according to specifications required by local building codes and ASHRAE standards. The engineer is likely to not understand what is required for healthy air. You may spend of lot of money paying for plans you can't use and have to re-do them yourself.

If the seams on air ducts are not sealed with mastic, air leaks into walls and ceilings and pressurizes those spaces. Air in the walls and ceilings is pushed into the living space.

Is There Ever Enough?

This was a new house, a green building so airtight only two windows can be opened—bedrooms in which code requires a fire escape. Knowing the house would be so airtight, the builder installed a mechanical ventilation system. Based on the square feet of the house, the builder calculated the amount of ventilation required by ASHRAE Standard 62.2 to be 50 cubic feet per minute (CFM). The builder decided the ventilator, capable of 100 CFM, only needed to be on half of the time and set it on a timer to run 12 hours a day.

I tested the air in the home. The laboratory tests results showed the total VOC was 7,600 nanograms per liter of air (ng/l). Leadership in Energy and Environmental Design (LEED) considers levels greater than 500 to be high.

After the first test results were poor, I increased the setting on the ventilator to 80 CFM and set it to run all the time. A few days later I re-tested the air. There was a 75% improvement. The level of VOCs was still high. Gas from the attached garage was a significant source. I suggested installing a bathroom fan in the garage to exhaust air from the garage 24/7.

I re-tested the air after the fan in the garage was installed. Installing the fan in the garage improved the air in the home as much as using the ventilator. Together, the ventilator (an ERV) and the fan in the garage (an ultra-quiet high volume, bathroom fan) reduced the total VOCs inside the home from 7,600 to 610 ng/l. To further improve the air, I recommended turning the CFM setting on the ventilator to its maximum, 100 CFM.

Builders are afraid to increase the amount of fresh air brought inside by ventilators. They build a house airtight. When it comes to ventilation, they kick and scream a house doesn't need *that* much. They don't know better.

The Alternatives

Size the air conditioner properly. It should run continuously. This is critical in hot and humid climates.

Install a ventilator(s) to bring in fresh air.

Install a big HEPA filter at the furnace or air-conditioner. The filter should be so big it requires it's own blower.

Choose between standard (flex) or metal ductwork.

Make sure the air ducts are sealed with mastic.

Have the ducts leak-tested before the insulation and drywall are installed. This can be done using the same machine that is used to measure how airtight a house is. The crew should pour theatrical fog into the machine as it pressurizes the ducts to make the leaks apparent.

Clothes dryers exhaust a lot of air. Consider installing a vent in the laundry room that goes through an outside wall and opens to provide make-up air into the laundry room when the dryer is running.

There is an issue with the kitchen range hood similar to the dryer. Consider you are cooking salmon for dinner, and it burns. You don't want the living room to smell like fish, so you turn the range hood on. With an airtight house (green building) it is going to be a slow and difficult process. It's going to take a long time for the smell to dissipate if there's no make-up air to help clear the air. There will be suction in the house as the hood tries to pull air through the attic and outside walls into the kitchen. A solution is to wire the hood to a vent on an exterior wall to open when the hood is turned on.

Recommendations

Install a Ventilator

Don't expect a single ventilator to make the air in a house healthy if there is more than one HVAC system. A ventilator only has the power of a large bathroom fan. One ventilator should be installed for every HVAC system.

Depending on the climate, choose an energy recovery ventilator (ERV) or heat recovery ventilator (HRV). Both transfer the heat between the outdoor air coming inside and the air being exhausted. ERVs also transfer humidity and are recommended in humid climates. As humid outdoor air comes inside, an ERV transfers the humidity to air being exhausted. This reduces the humidity of the air brought inside. ERVs cost more than HRVs.

Choose a brand. Manufacturers include Panasonic®, Lifebreath®, and Broan®. Ventilators should be 4-duct systems. Two-duct systems are less effective. Stock filters should be upgraded to MERV 10 or HEPA if it's an option.

Choose a size (CMF). Bigger is better. Use the ASHRAE standard to check what the <u>minimum</u> ventilation rate should be based on the square footage of the home. ASHRAE assumes 8-foot-high ceilings. If the house has high ceilings, take that into consideration. At least twice the ASHRAE recommendation is required to have healthy air in the home.

Because the materials in ventilators off-gas styrofoam and plastic, order ventilators when construction begins. When they arrive, remove them from the boxes and store them out of the packaging so they can air out.

Design Blueprints for the Ventilation System

1. Ask the builder for a clean, legible floor plan that notes where the builder would like to locate the ventilators. Ventilators should be located inside closets in the occupied space. Do not put ventilators in the attic. Do not put them in mechanical closets in which there are gas appliances. They can be put in a closet next to a mechanical

closet if the closet door is weather-stripped.

2. Get two colored ink markers. Use green to specify the fresh-air vents and supply air ducts; use red to specify the return air vents and return air ducts.

3. Mark on the floor plan where in each room a supply vent is desired. Each room that has an HVAC supply vent should also have a fresh-air vent from a ventilator. To avoid drafts and discomfort, supply vents should not be located directly over a bed, sitting area, or desk. Supply vents should not be located in kitchens or bathrooms. Bedrooms, living rooms, and offices should have supply vents. Vents may be placed on the ceiling.

4. Each room that has a fresh-air supply vent should also have a return vent. The return vent should be at the opposite side of the room, 10 feet or more from the supply vent. Using red ink, mark where the return air vents will be. They may be on the ceiling.

If it is not possible to install a return vent in a room with a supply vent, a return air pathway register should be installed in the wall between the room and hallway. In that case it's likely the builder is suggesting a common return vent in the hallway (not recommended). Return air pathway registers dampen sound and light transmissions for privacy while allowing air to flow from one side of the wall to the other. Without a pathway register, less fresh air will flow into the room. This affects heating and cooling as well as ventilation.

5. Using green ink, draw a straight line from each supply vent to connect it to the ventilator. These are the fresh-air ducts. Try to make the lines as straight as possible and avoid turns.

6. Draw in red, a line from each return vent to connect it to the ventilator. These are the return air ducts. Return air ducts may run side-by-side with supply air ducts as they approach a ventilator.

7. Using green ink, draw a straight line from the ventilator to an exterior wall at which the fresh-air duct to the outside will be installed. It should be on the side of the house, below the roofline, and not near a gas meter or trash cans. This line should be as short and straight as possible. If it is long (50 feet or more) or requires a 90-degree turn, consider an alternative location for the ventilator closet. Try to get the ventilator as close to an outside wall as possible. The fresh-air vent should not be on the roof.

8. The exhaust from the ventilator to the outside should go straight up to the roof. There's no need to mark this on the plan.

9. An exhaust fan should be installed in the garage with a minimum of 80 CFM for each bay. It should run continuously. Draw in red where the fan should be on the

ceiling in the garage. Draw a line from it to an outside wall.

10. Give the marked up plan to the builder and request that the ventilators, vents, and air ducts be installed where noted.

11. Consider soundproofing the interior walls around closets in which there are ventilators. This can be done installing cellulose or wool batt insulation inside the walls. Do not use fiberglass.

Specify the Materials

The fresh-air supply duct feeding a ventilator should be metal. A short section of flexible duct may be used to connect metal ducts to the ventilator. The return air ducts can also be metal.

To prevent condensation, metal ducts should be insulated on the outside using foil-faced R-8 fiberglass insulation sleeves or equivalent.

Tell the Builder

Tell the builder the following:

• The ventilators should run all the time, at the maximum CFM rate they are capable of. Do not set them on timers.

- Do not reduce the CFM of fresh air based on calculations in *ASHRAE Standard 62.2.*

- Dampers should not be placed inside ventilation ducts. Dampers malfunction. If code requires one, a backdraft damper may be installed on the outside of the building where the duct terminates. This allows it to be visually inspected to verify that it opens and closes properly.

- Ducts for the ventilator should not have volume control dampers. These malfunction. A damper is not required as the CFM will be set to 100%.

Heating and Air-Conditioning

For a HEPA filter, a Pure Air Systems Model 600HS Plus is recommended. I have measured it using a laser-particle counter, and it's a true HEPA. It needs to be installed in tandem with the furnace and air-conditioning systems. The HEPA filter is so thick it has its own blower to push air though it. There is an option to add carbon to remove odors and formaldehyde.

An outdoor air intake can be connected to the Pure Air Systems filter in a manner such that the furnace or air-conditioner can be used for ventilation when it's running. To do this, connect a four-inch duct from outside to the HEPA. When the furnace or air conditioner runs, it will pull fresh air into the filter, and the house will be

What Your Builder Should Know

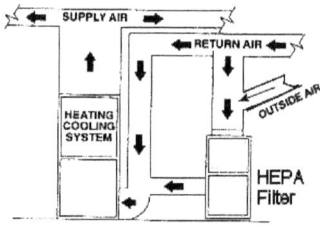

pressurized with fresh air the same way a commercial building is. This is not a substitute for having a separate ventilation system as it only works when the furnace or air-conditioner is running.

Use metal for ductwork. Metal is easier to clean and does not off-gas plastic. Place the insulation on the OUTSIDE of the metal ducts. Do not allow metal ducts to be manufactured by gluing insulation to the inside of them, the common method.

Give This to Your Builder

05 05 00 COMMON WORK RESULTS FOR METALS

Sheet metal ductwork should be cleaned before it is installed using a high-pressure hose and acceptable cleaning product. T.S.P. may be used.

23 01 00 OPERATION AND MAINTENANCE OF HVAC SYSTEMS

The HVAC vents and return openings should be sealed and not used for heating or cooling during construction.

23 05 66 ANTIMICROBIAL ULTRAVIOLET EMITTERS FOR HVAC

In humid climates, install a UV light to shine on the coils inside the air-conditioner. This inhibits the growth of bacteria that cause musty odors. It's only effective if it shines on the coils.

23 31 00 HVAC DUCTS

Duct board and flex type ducts should not be used. Use metal for ducts. Place the insulation on the OUTSIDE of the metal ducts. Do not allow metal ducts to be manufactured by gluing an insulation liner to the inside of the ducts.

HVAC systems and ducts should not be placed in attics, a crawlspace, or a garage. Furnaces and ductwork should be located within the conditioned living space with access for changing filters.

Duct seams shall be sealed with a water-based approved mastic.

A duct blaster inspection should be performed to pressure check the ductwork and seal leaks before closing walls and ceilings with insulation and drywall. Leaks should be identified and repaired with the aid of theatrical fog.

23 32 00 AIR PLENUMS

Wall cavities and building plenums shall not be used as air ducts, including where an HVAC unit attaches to the return. Ductwork shall not be located in exterior walls or under concrete slabs.

23 34 00 HVAC FANS

HVAC systems shall be sized for the space based on calculations following ACCA Manual J and Manual D. Request contractors provide calculations with their bids.

Fiberglass and materials used for insulation, sound reduction, or acoustics shall not be exposed to the air stream inside the blower. Materials such as these should be covered with foil and foil tape.

Fan compartment doors shall have a gasket.

What Your Builder Should Know

23 35 00 1 EXHAUST FANS

Exhaust fans shall be quiet, less than 1.0 sone.

23 35 00 2 MAKE-UP AIR FOR LAUNDRY ROOM

Install a through-the-wall (exterior wall) ventilator in the laundry room to provide make-up air when the dryer is running. The vent should be wired to open when the dryer is running. Examples are the Honeywell Fresh Air Ventilation System and Control and products made by CCB Innovations. HEPA filtration is not an issue. The dryer will use the outdoor air being pulled in. This contains and isolates the air in the laundry room and prevents the air pressure in the house from going negative (less than outside) when the dryer runs.

23 35 00 3 EXHAUST FAN IN GARAGE

Install an exhaust fan(s) in the garage with a minimum of 80 CFM per bay, set to run continuously, exhausted outside. The switch controlling the fan should be labeled with instructions to leave it on. The fan shall be the quiet, less than 0.5 sone.

23 37 13 DIFFUSERS, REGISTERS, AND GRILLES

Install a pass-through grill vent in each room that has a supply vent but no return vent.

23 41 00 PARTICULATE AIR FILTRATION

Leave room in the mechanical closet for installing a Pure Air Systems model 600HS Plus. The Pure Air Systems system has its own blower and is connected to the HVAC in by-pass configuration. Install a fresh-air intake from outside into the return side of the Pure Air Systems unit. The intake should have a normally closed and sealed spring damper and critter screen. Reference the manufacturer's drawings.

Ventilation and HVAC

23 42 00 GAS-PHASE AIR FILTRATION

Activated carbon and other media are options with Pure Air Systems for removing odors and formaldehyde. The owner may order and install these as required. Ensure there is access to change the filters.

23 72 23 PACKAGED AIR-TO-AIR ENERGY RECOVERY UNITS (VENTILATORS)

Bathroom fans or the kitchen range hood shall not be used as ventilation systems. Bathroom fans and the range exhaust shall be dedicated to source control.

An ERV or HRV ventilator shall be installed. A separate ventilator with dedicated ductwork shall be installed for each HVAC system.

Order the ventilators when the project begins so that they have time to off-gas. They should be taken out of the boxes and unpackaged when they arrive and left to sit in a clean environment until they are installed.

Do not reduce the rate of fresh air (CMF) on a ventilator based on calculations in ASHRAE Standard 62.2. Use the standard to determine the minimum ventilation required. At least twice that amount is required to have low VOCs and healthy air in a home. The controls on the ventilator should be set to bring in the maximum amount of outdoor air and run 24/7.

Dampers should not be placed inside air ducts. If a damper malfunctions, it can be difficult to diagnose and repair, resulting in less fresh air. If code requires it, a backdraft damper may be installed on the outside of the building where it can be periodically checked and serviced if necessary.

The ducts for the ventilator should not have volume control dampers. These can malfunction. A damper is not required as we intend to set the CFM for outdoor air at 100%.

The controls on the ventilator may be set to slightly pressurize a house, bringing in more fresh air than what is exhausted. The exception is in cold climates, for which an equal amount of air shall be specified.

A supply vent should be installed in each bedroom and sitting area where an HVAC duct is installed. The supply vent should not be located directly over a bed, sitting area, or desk. Provide the owner with a floor plan. Ask the owner to mark on the floor plan where in each room a supply vent and a return vent to the ventilator are desired.

A return vent should be installed at the opposite end of each room in which a supply vent is installed. For rooms with a supply vent, without a return vent, a return air pathway register shall be installed. These dampen sound and light transmission and allow air to flow from one side of the wall to the other. This allows air to flow from these rooms to the central return.

The exhaust for the ventilator should be on the roof and not close to a sewer or plumbing vent.

The main fresh-air supply duct feeding a ventilator should be metal, as straight as possible, and close to an exterior wall to reduce the length of the run. It should not have elbows or turns that will reduce the amount of fresh air brought in. A short section of flexible duct may be used to connect the duct to a ventilator. The fresh-air intake for the ventilator should be on the side of the house and not near a dryer vent, kitchen range exhaust, or gas utility meter. It should not be on the same side of the house that garbage cans will be stored. It should not be on the roof.

An outdoor air intake shall be installed in the kitchen to prevent the air pressure in the house from becoming negative (less than outside) when the range hood is turned on. Example products are the Broan SmartSense® Fan Automatic Make-Up Air Damper and products by CCB Innovations. These consist of two parts. A sensor is installed in the hood exhaust duct. It is wired to open a damper installed in an exterior wall. The outdoor vent should come through an exterior wall, pass under a kitchen cabinet, and terminate at the kick plate on one side of the stove. The intent is to prevent outdoor air from competing with cooking gases needing to be exhausted. The outdoor air should mix with ambient air in the kitchen before being pulled into the exhaust. If there is a pantry, and the pantry does not have a door, the duct may be installed in the pantry.

Ventilation and HVAC

One builder suggested to bring in the make-up air for the dryer and kitchen range through an outside air duct connected to the air conditioning and heating system. The issue is there will not be make-up air unless the blower in the air conditioning or heating system is running. If it seems like a bad idea to dump hot air into a kitchen, consider where the make-up air for the kitchen range and dryer come in a normal house - from outside, through leaks in walls, around windows, doors, the attic—hot places. There are high levels of particulates in a kitchen air while cooking. If the hood needs to be turned on, the ambient air in the kitchen has a higher particulate count than outdoors. HEPA filtration is not required for make-up air. Keep it simple—use a product wired to the hood and dryer to open the outdoor vents when the hood or dryer is turned on. Avoid complicated make-up air systems with variable fan speeds that try to control the amount of air let in. These can malfunction and may be more expensive.

23 76 00 EVAPORATIVE AIR-COOLING EQUIPMENT

Evaporative coolers are a healthy and effective way to cool a house and introduce fresh outdoor air. Use pads that have not been treated and do not have an odor. Most pads have foul odors from ammonium used in the antimicrobial. New pads may not have an odor until they get wet. Test the product by soaking it in water and smelling it before installing in the swamp cooler.

23 81 26 SPLIT-SYSTEM AIR-CONDITIONERS

For soundproofing, do not put a compressor for a split-package air-conditioner outside next to a bedroom or sitting area.

23 84 00 HUMIDITY CONTROL EQUIPMENT

In humid climates, an Aprilaire® Ultra-Aire Whole House Dehumidifier or similar system should be installed to aid with dehumidification. One or two units may be needed depending on the size of the house. The outdoor air shall go into the Aprilaire® (or similar system) and exhaust into the return of the HVAC.

What Your Builder Should Know

Framing

What It Is

The walls and roof are put on.

After the local building department inspects the framing, the builder will cover it with plywood to make exterior walls and the roof. Oriented strand board (OSB) or an alternative type of sheathing may be used. Holes are cut for doors and windows.

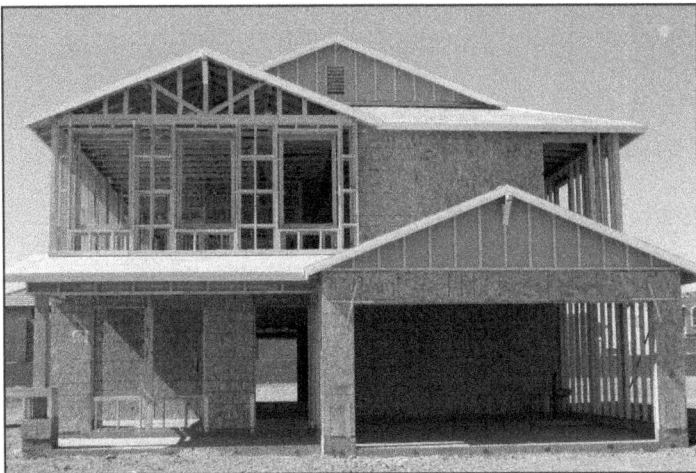

What Your Builder Should Know

Some homes have a stone facade, behind which there is a brick or wood framed wall. The stone, adhered manufactured stone veneer, is manufactured by mixing cement with color pigments. The framed walls and weather barrier behind the stone must be constructed to prevent water from leaking into the house.

Categories of Concern

Mold
EMFs

Shortcuts and Standard Practices

Most builders accept wood as delivered. They don't inspect it for mold and may expect it to be wet. Upon receiving it, they don't cover it to protect it from rain and snow.

What Can Go Wrong Here

Wood may arrive damp or moldy.

Wood may get wet if uncovered, and it rains before the roof is put on. Mold can grow if a period of rain persists. The general consensus is three or four days of moisture is sufficient for mold to start growing. A preventative solution is to tent the house until the roof is on. I have never seen this done.

A builder may treat the framing with an antimicrobial or paint it with an antimicrobial paint. This does not remove mold. Although labels on antimicrobial treatments say they are non-toxic, the treatments leave residual chemicals and biocides. A common residual is alkaline copper quaternary ammonium.

Leaks and damage can occur if the stone veneer is not installed correctly.

The Alternatives

One way to have mold-free lumber is to specify kiln-dried wood. It's expensive. Older houses were built with it. The wood must be kept dry before the roof is put on, otherwise it may be wasted money.

Treated lumber is used on the bottom piece of a framed wall to prevent it from rotting if the wood gets wet. The healthiest, least toxic type of wood treatment is made with boric acid. Boric acid also prevents termites. The acid inhibits digestive enzymes, causing termites to starve. PACBOR® is a line of wood products treated with boric acid. Bora-Care® is a liquid applied by spraying. It may be used on wood, OSB, and wood composite materials. Builders can obtain LEED® points for using it.

If you don't use borates your contractor will use what

is available. It's likely to be alkaline copper quaternary (ACQ) or copper azole (CA). ACQ may have a slight ammonia odor. CA contains triazole herbicides that are carcinogenic.

Treated wood is traditionally green. The green color is due to the copper used to inhibit fungal growth. New formulations require less copper, and the wood may not be green. Red dye may be added to make wood look like redwood.

OSB is the type of sheathing commonly used for exterior walls. Don't use it. Specify CDX plywood for subfloors, walls, and the roof decking. If plywood gets wet, it takes longer for mold to grow compared to OSB. AdvanTech™ plywood, made water-resistant by adding polyurethane, is another alternative.

Bedrooms are good places to soundproof. Soundproofing is done similar to how firewalls are constructed: frame two separate walls, back to back, with the studs alternated, leaving a space between them that is filled with cellulose or mineral wool insulation.

Recommendations

Prohibit OSB. Specify plywood. The highest quality, most expensive types of plywood are A & B grades. The economical grades are C & D. Use CDX plywood for exterior walls and roofs. "X" does not stand for exterior. It

Framing

stands for exposure. CDX can withstand some moisture. One side is grade C, the other D. The two sides are bonded with glue that can withstand moisture.

Do not allow the builder to treat wood with an antimicrobial or encapsulate (paint) it to cover mold.

Use a moisture meter to check wood as it is delivered. Send damp or moldy wood back to the supplier. Store wood to keep it dry. Create a moisture management plan and keep it on-site. It should state the following:

- Do not accept damp wood (moisture readings of 19% or higher) or water-damaged wood (stained or discolored.)

- Store wood covered on a pallet, even if it's sunny.

- If it rains before the roof is on, and the framing is not dry in two days, stop work and bring in fans to expedite drying the wood framing. If visible mold or staining is present, stop work and clean the wood after it is dry (less than 19%). Lightly sandblast the wood. A wire-brush or sander may be used. If a significant amount of wood has mold, consider cleaning it using dry ice blasting. Pellets of dry ice are abrasive and clean the wood. The pellets, made of carbon dioxide, evaporate after being used. Sandblasting makes a mess and is not recommended. Soda blasting is not recommended.

- Do not enclose the walls with insulation and dry-wall if the moisture readings of wood are greater than 19%.

Check for This

As wood is delivered, verify it is clean, dry, and free of mold. Check the wood with a moisture meter. Do not accept wood with readings greater than 19%. Make sure the builder has designated a place to store wood to be covered and protected from rain and snow.

Give This to Your Builder

01 35 13 WOOD MANAGEMENT PLAN

Wood should be stored in a manner to keep it dry. Elevate it off the ground and cover it with a tarp. Do not completely seal the tarp. Allow for ventilation on all sides.

Wall and floor framing should not be enclosed if the moisture content of the framing exceeds 19%.

If it rains after wood is installed, moisture readings should be taken. If readings of framed wood, subflooring or sheathing exceed 19% for more than two days, fans shall be used to expedite drying to less than 19%. The wood shall be inspected for mold when it is dry (<19%). Mold, if present, shall be removed by mechanical means: wire-brushing and sanding, in accordance with the *S520 Standard for Professional Mold Remediation.* Under no circumstances shall wood be treated for mold or encapsulated (painted to cover or treat mold).

Framing

01 65 00 PRODUCT DELIVERY REQUIREMENTS
01 65 05 WOOD INSPECTION

Wood being delivered shall be inspected and found to be free of mold and water damage. Wood with signs of water damage (staining) or mold shall be refused for delivery.

The moisture content of wood shall be measured as it is delivered using the penetrating pins on a moisture meter. The moisture content shall be at or below 19%. Wood that does not meet this requirement shall be refused for delivery or returned to the supplier. Readings shall be recorded in a logbook with the date and delivery details. According to the *IICRC Standard for Professional Water Damage Restoration*, the normal moisture content of dry wood is at or below 16%; between 17 % and 19% is considered damp; 20% or greater is considered wet.

01 66 05 WOOD STORAGE AND MANAGEMENT

Wood should be stored in a manner to keep it dry by elevating it off the ground, cross stacking it on a pallet, and covering it with a tarp. Do not seal the tarp. Allow for ventilation on all sides.

If the moisture content of wood goes above 19%, wood shall be dried by cross stacking on a pallet in a sheltered location and using fans. Wood shall be inspected for mold when readings indicate dry conditions, less than or equal to 19%.

06 05 73 WOOD TREATMENT

The client will specify acceptable and non-acceptable products for treating wood. Unfinished structural lumber may be treated with Bora-Care®. It contains boric acid, comes as a liquid that is mixed with water, and is applied by spraying.

ACCEPTABLE WOOD ADHESIVES

Use Elmer's® Carpenter's Wood Glue for finish carpentry and cabinets. Use 100% silicone caulk as a subfloor adhesive.

06 13 00 Heavy Timber Construction

Large diameter log and viga-style beams should be air-dried, the process of letting wood dry covered in open air. Air-drying allows for even drying. Wood should be stored and protected from rain.

06 14 00 Treated Wood Foundations

The following are prohibited:

- creosote
- pentachlorophenol
- chromated copper arsenate (CCA)
- ammoniated copper arsenic (ACA)

Acceptable:

- wood treated with Bora-Care®
- PACBOR®, wood treated with boric acid
- alkaline copper quaternary (ACQ)
- copper azole (CA)
- micronized copper (MCA or MCQ)

06 16 01 Exterior Sheathing

Plywood should be purchased in advance and stacked to allow airflow while being protected from moisture.

The following are unacceptable:

- products containing asphalt
- paper-faced drywall
- foam insulation board
- pressure-treated plywood

The following are acceptable:

- CDX plywood
- exterior-grade plywood
- AdvanTech™

06 15 33 WOOD PATIO DECKING

Acceptable products include:

- redwood
- Trex®, planks made from saw dust and recycled plastic
- ipe (e-pay), a hard wood resistant to mold

06 16 23 SUBFLOORING

The following are unacceptable:

- pressboard
- orientated strand board (OSB)
- products containing asphalt
- pressure-treated plywood

The following are acceptable:

- CDX plywood
- exterior-grade plywood
- AdvanTech™
- structural cementitious sheeting

06 16 26 UNDERLAYMENT

If requested, non-asphalt underlayments include:

- Titanium® UD
- RoofTopGuard II
- Tyvek® Supro

06 16 26.1 ICE DAMMING

In cold climates, a self-adhering roofing underlayment, such as Ice & Water Shield®, should be installed. Local code may require installing it six feet up from the edge of a roof. Install it on the entire roof.

06 16 26.2 ROOF SHEATHING

The following are acceptable:

• tongue and groove (solid wood)
• CDX-grade plywood
• AdvanTech™

Weatherproofing, Doors, and Windows

What It Is

After plywood or another type of sheathing is installed to create the outside walls and the roof, the house is wrapped to protect it from rain and moisture. The traditional material used to weatherproof houses is asphalt-impregnated (tar) building paper. Mold can't grow on surfaces treated with tar.

In order to make houses airtight, green builders use housewrap instead of building paper. Housewrap is less effective in preventing moisture intrusion and mold than building paper.

After the building paper or housewrap is installed, the builder will install the windows and exterior doors. Doors and windows are included in this section because mistakes are made weatherproofing around doors and windows. It's rare to find a house that is weatherproofed properly around doors and windows.

Categories of Concern

Mold
Light

Shortcuts and Standard Practices

Contractors often install housewrap around the windows first and install windows before the rest of the house is wrapped. Mistakes happen when the remainder of the house is wrapped, and water leaks inside.

What Can Go Wrong Here

Housewrap works well to make houses airtight; it's less effective at weatherproofing and keeping water out. Using two layers of traditional building paper is the best way to weatherproof a house.

Most builders don't know how to flash a window properly. Exterior doors are often not flashed.

Windows have labels to help choose ones best suited for a location in the home and climate. Contractors looking for the cheapest windows may overlook such labels without consulting the homeowner. It may be too hot or bright in a room.

Weatherproofing

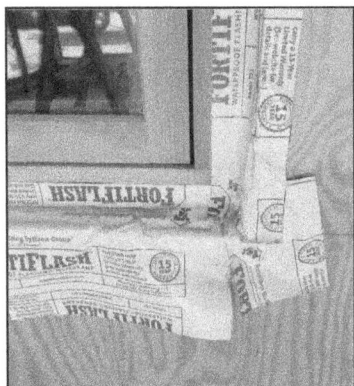

Figure 1: An example of how NOT to flash a window. The builder thought the idea was to keep water out. He didn't consider where water goes if the window leaks.

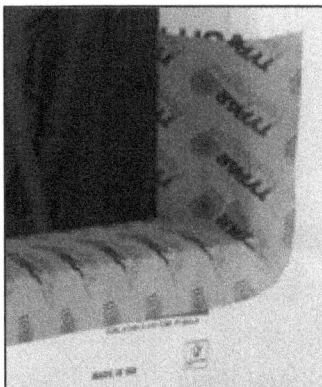

Figure 2: An example of how to flash a window CORRECTLY. The flashing should seal the opening before the window is inserted.

The term housewrap is used here as generic descriptor. Housewrap® and Tyvek® are registered trademarks for high-density polyethylene (HDPE) vapor and air barriers. In theory, housewrap is like Gore-Tex®—vapor (sweat) can pass through, air and water (wind and rain) cannot. The belief is housewrap can be used to make a house airtight and at the same time waterproof. But consider what happened if you wear a Gore-Tex® rain jacket without a shirt. Imagine the jacket is pressed tight against your bare skin. It becomes wet and uncomfortable. It's the same with housewrap. Housewrap is stapled to the plywood sheathing. Water trapped behind housewrap cannot dry out. The wood will stay wet, grow mold, and rot. Housewrap is not a good material to use if you are concerned about mold and moisture.

In 2002, I ordered a book called *The Moisture Control Handbook*. It came with a note from Joseph Lstiburek, one of the authors. It said:

> The Moisture Control Handbook was published in 1993. In the past decade several things have become obvious to me that are not reflected adequately in the Handbook. The most significant is the role of polyethylene (housewrap) on retarding the drying of building assemblies. I have come to the conclusion that polyethylene is really a "drying retarder" and should be avoided.

Polyethylene (housewrap) has plasticizers and additives added to make it strong and soft, rather than hard and brittle, and for UV protection. There may be emissions of plasticizers inside walls at warm temperatures. Odors inside have not been reported. Building paper off-gases trace amounts of hydrogen sulfide inside walls at temperatures above 120 F. Odors inside a home have not been reported.

Weatherproofing

Rain Story

In a new house, in a new development, I did a mold inspection for the buyer. It was dry, and the house looked perfect. My client purchased the home. A week later it rained. He called me, saying water was leaking under several of the windows. I told him water could not leak inside if the windows were flashed correctly. The builder assured him the windows had been flashed correctly. I told the builder to verify this by removing a window.

The builder removed a window and found the windows had been flashed improperly. The builder offered to buy the house back. The following day the builder changed his mind as he realized the windows had been flashed the wrong way in all of the new homes in the development. Instead of removing the windows the builder decided to remove the siding around the windows and install additional flashing over the edges of the windows (Figure 1), something that does not prevent water from leaking inside. The buyer gave up the dispute and paid out of pocket to have the windows removed and flashed properly.

The Alternatives

If local code requires housewrap, use housewrap and traditional building paper. Wrap the house first with a layer of housewrap, and then install a layer of building paper over the housewrap. If code does not require using housewrap, do not use it. Install two layers of Grade D building paper instead.

Recommendations

Read the labels on windows to find the best combination of light emitted and UV blocked. Wood is the best choice for window cladding.

If code requires housewrap, install a layer of traditional building paper over the housewrap. If code does not require housewrap, install two layers of building paper.

Make sure the windows are not installed until all the sheathing (plywood or OSB), housewrap, and building paper is installed.

Make sure the windows are flashed using a peel-and-stick, self-adhering membrane. Ask the builder to flash one window first and allow you it inspect it before the rest of the windows are installed. Ask for pictures or video of the crew flashing windows at another house. Do this before construction begins so there is time to discuss how the windows should be flashed.

Avoid decorative glass block windows, the type installed in bathrooms. These are difficult to flash and often not flashed by the builder.

Weatherproofing

Custom doors can be made healthier than factory-made as they allow healthier finishes to be used.

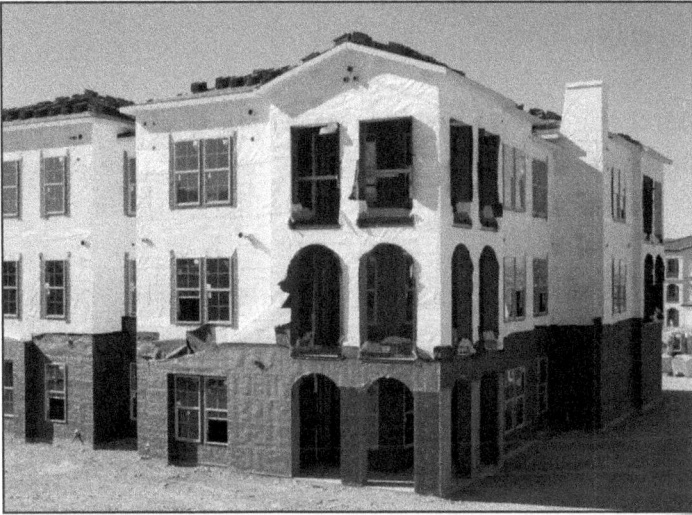

The best of both worlds. Housewrap was put on first. A layer of building paper is being installed, shingle fashion, bottom to top, over the housewrap. It would have been preferable if the building paper was installed over the housewrap before the windows were installed.

Check for This

After the framing is completed, BEFORE the ply-wood or OSB sheathing is put on, inspect the framing for mold. If mold is visible, stop work. The simplest method of removing mold may be sandblasting. A light blasting is sufficient. A leaf blower should be used afterwards to blow dust off the wood and out of the house. Sometimes it's only few pieces of wood that are moldy. If it's an isolated occurrence, the builder may be happy to replace them.

After the housewrap is installed, BEFORE the windows are installed, inspect the housewrap for tears. Tears should be mended using the housewrap tape.

Ask the builder to have one window flashed before the rest and allow you to inspect it to make sure it was flashed correctly. Do not wait until all of the windows are installed to notify the builder there is an issue with the way the windows are flashed. There is an easy way to tell if a window is flashed correctly—the bottom window flange and the nails on the bottom flange should be visible.

Give This to Your Builder

02 87 13 Mold Remediation

If required, mold remediation shall be performed according to *IICRC S520 Standard for Professional Mold Remediation.* Mold needs to be physically removed by sanding, brushing, and cleaning. Antimicrobials and encapsulants are prohibited for reasons explained in the standard.

07 27 19 Plastic Sheet Air Barrier

If local code requires using housewrap, install a layer of building paper on top of the housewrap before the windows are installed. If housewrap is not required, install two layers of Grade D building paper. Two layers are shown to provide better drainage control than one layer behind all types of cladding.

An inspection of the housewrap shall be made before installing windows and doors. Tears shall be mended using housewrap tape.

07 62 00 SHEET METAL FLASHING AND TRIM

Ensure all of the proper flashing is installed. This includes primary and secondary (roof return) kick-out flashing, step flashing, chimney cap flashing, saddles, and crickets next to skylights and chimneys.

07 65 00 FLEXIBLE FLASHING

Windows should be flashed using a peel-and-stick, self-adhering membrane. The flashing needs to be the depth of the windowsill plus a few inches to lap down the exterior wall, over the housewrap or building paper. For example, if the framing is 2x6, a flashing membrane of nine inches is required.

Exterior doors should be flashed using a self-adhering membrane.

INSTRUCTIONS FOR FLASHING WINDOWS:

Do not install window flashing until all of the sheathing, building paper, and housewrap are installed.

For recessed windows, the entire window opening should be flashed, with the flashing extending over and on top of the housewrap (or building paper) on all sides before inserting the window.

For windows flush with the exterior sheathing, the procedure is as follows. Use a flexible, peel-and-stick flashing. The flashing needs to be the depth of the windowsill plus a few inches to lap down the exterior wall, over the housewrap or building paper. For example, if the framing is 2x6, a flashing membrane of nine inches is required.

What Your Builder Should Know

1. Cut a hole in the building paper or housewrap and fold it back.

2. Place a sill pan on the windowsill. Manufactured pan-flashing systems include the Weathermate™ by Dow®.

3. Install flashing over the pan and up the framing on each side of the window to the top of the window. Lap the flashing over the building paper and/or housewrap. The flashing should extend over the front edge of the windowsill and overlap the building paper and/or housewrap by three inches.

5. Caulk behind the top and side flanges of the window, taking care to cover nail holes. Do not caulk the bottom flange. Water needs to escape out the bottom.

6. Insert the window. Nail or screw the window in place. Do not spray foam between the framing and the window for insulation or to make it airtight. Foam is not waterproof and interferes with drainage.

7. Install flashing on each side of the window, extending a few inches above and below the window. The peel-and-stick should go over the housewrap building paper on each side of the window. Use a roller to press the flashing tight against the building to ensure a good bond.

8. Apply peel-and-stick flashing across the top of the window, lapping it across the peel-and-sticks that were applied on each side.

9. Caulk across the top of the window frame.

10. After caulking, install a piece of metal Z-flashing on the window header to push water dripping down out, over the front edge of the window.

11. Apply a layer of peel-and-stick across the top of the Z-flashing.

12. Pull down the housewrap building paper over the Z-flashing onto the top of the window.

13. Tape the housewrap building paper on top of the window to keep it in place over the Z-flashing. Do not tape all the way

across. Skip parts to allow water dripping down to escape and not collect behind the tape.

Peel-and-stick flashing <u>does not</u> go under the bottom of the window after the window is in place.

Caulk does not go under the bottom of the window. Water needs to be able to drip out the bottom.

08 05 00 COMMON WORK RESULTS FOR OPENINGS

Door Thresholds

Exterior doors should be sealed under the threshold with silicon.

A metal pan flashing should be installed under exterior door thresholds. The pan should slope down from the grade of the finished floor, under the door, and lap down the outside of the foundation.

Doors between the garage and living space should be sealed under the threshold with silicon caulk.

Weather Stripping

Doors between the living space and garage shall be weather sealed.

Doors between the living space and mechanical rooms shall be weather sealed.

8 10 00 DOORS AND FRAMES

When exterior doors arrive, remove the metal bottom pieces and caulk between the bottom piece and the door.

For soundproofing, caulk between doorjambs and framing as interior doors are installed at bedrooms.

What Your Builder Should Know

08 14 00 WOOD DOORS

To prevent off-gassing, manufactured doors should be sealed. Use an approved sealant, GREENGUARD certified, or a product from AFM Safecoat® on all sides.

8 60 00 ROOF WINDOWS AND SKYLIGHTS

Require the manufacturer of roof windows and skylights to provide drawings showing how roof windows and skylights will be flashed.

8 80 00 GLAZING

Windows should be selected based on Energy Star ratings in regard to visible light transmittance, reflectance, solar gain, and shading. This will vary depending on where the windows are installed in the house and the function of the room.

Siding

What It Is

Siding is installed. This may include vinyl, wood, stone veneer, stucco, metal, shingles, and other types of claddings.

Categories of Concern

Mold

Shortcuts and Standard Practices

Water that gets behind siding needs a way out. Weep holes and exits at the bottom of siding on exterior walls are often missing or covered by paint, stucco, or mortar. If there is not a way for water to get out, water will build up and leak inside.

What Can Go Wrong Here

The proper flashing may not be installed around doors,

windows, or on the roof.

The Alternatives

The choice of exterior siding often depends on what's normal for the geographic location. For stucco, avoid acrylic-based synthetic stucco coating. These trap moisture and cause the finish to bubble. Use traditional, cement-based stucco. For the details on how stucco should terminate as it reaches the ground and the top of the slab, have your builder reference, *Best Practices Guide to Residential Construction: Materials, Finishes, and Details* by Steven Bliss.

For brick, make sure the mason creates weep holes at a course of brick a few courses from the ground. Leave gaps in the mortar on the sides of a few bricks so that water that gets behind the brick wall can drain out as it reaches the ground.

For stone veneer, make sure the builder follows the guidelines in *Installation Guide and Detailing Options for Compliance with ASTM C1780 For Adhered Manufactured Stone Veneer* by The Masonry Veneer Manufacturers Association. The most common places leaks occur are around doors and windows. This guide contains drawings and details on how stone should be installed and sealed around doors and windows.

Siding

Check for This

Before the siding is installed, make sure the windows are flashed correctly. It helps to think like you're a drop of rainwater. Starting from the top of the wall over a window, imagine you are dripping down. Is there a way you can get into the house? If so, there is a better way to install the flashing around the windows. If so, the windows need to be removed to flash them effectively.

After the siding is installed, check there is a minimum of two inches of clearance between the bottom of the siding and hard surfaces (driveways, porches, sidewalks) and four inches between the bottom of the siding and soft grade (landscaping). The bottom of the siding should have weep holes or be screed to allow water behind the siding to exit as it reaches the ground.

Give This to Your Builder

All sidings should be installed with the proper methods of transition and sealant between the siding and doors, the windows, the trim, the roof, and the foundation, according to specifications by the manufacturer and those published by the industry. This includes using weep screeds and backer rods as needed. It includes caulking around penetrations such as electrical outlets, light fixtures, overflow pipes, gas pipes, conduits, hose spigots, doors, and windows.

9 24 23 CEMENT STUCCO

Use two layers of 30-minute or 60-minute Grade D building paper. Two layers are specified since stucco tends to stick to the outer layer. A drainage space is created in the gap between the two layers. The wetter the climate, the heavier the building paper should be. In coastal areas contractors use two layers of 60-minute paper.

Do not apply stucco when it's hot or below 40 F. The scratch coat should be cured for 48 hours, during which it is kept damp by misting. Forty-eight hours later, the brown coat should be installed. The brown coat should be cured for 7 to 14 days.

Weep screeds with drain holes should be installed at the bottom of stucco walls. The stucco should terminate four inches above ground. The stucco company and painter need to prevent covering the weep holes.

Parapets should have metal caps. A waterproof self-adhering membrane should be installed under the cap. The cap should extend, sloping downward, two inches over the top of the parapet wall.

Vertical expansion joints shall be installed every ten feet.

Floor line expansion joints shall be installed between floors.

Roofing

What It Is

After vent pipes and any chimneys are installed, it's time to install the roofing shingles, tile, or a metal roof.

Categories of Concern

Mold

What Can Go Wrong Here

The roofer may not have installed the appropriate flashing or did it incorrectly. Typical weak points are around chimneys, skylights, the edge of a roof, valleys where two sections of roofs meet, and the edge of a roof where it touches a wall on a side of the house.

If you live in a cold climate, melting snow can back up under the roof at the edge, resulting in what's called ice damming. As water from melting snow reaches the edge of the roof, it re-freezes, blocking further water from getting off the roof. Water backs up and leaks into the house.

The Alternatives

Design with an abundance of portals and porches. Short overhangs over doors and windows help prevent mold by keeping water from wind and driving rain off vulnerable locations.

Do not have a flat roof. If you a flat roof, use a thermoplastic olefin (TPO) membrane as the roofing material.

Recommendations

Find a good roofer to install the roof. Ask the roofer to provide drawings and details regarding the types of flashing your type of construction should have.

In cold climates, install a membrane, such as Ice & Water Shield®, at the edge of the roof. Some homeowners install it on the entire roof.

Check for This

After the underlayment (felt building paper) is installed, before the roofing tiles or shingles are installed, inspect for flashing. This is technical. Find a roofer or home inspector to go with you who is knowledgeable about flashing. Check chimneys, dormers, valleys, skylights, sidewalls for kick out flashing, and above doors and windows.

Give This to Your Builder

Ensure the roofer installs the proper flashing. This includes around and next to dormers, valleys, skylights, doors, and windows. Kick-out flashing should be installed where a section of the roof touches a sidewall. Chimneys should have metal caps and crickets. Skylights should have crickets to divert water.

In climates with snow, a peel-and-stick underlayment, such as Ice & Water Shield®, should be installed a minimum of six feet up from the edge of the roof. Ask the client if they want it to be installed on the entire roof.

07 54 00 THERMOPLASTIC MEMBRANE ROOFING (FOR FLAT ROOFS)

Install a thermoplastic polyolefin (TPO) membrane. Choose a thickness resistant to punctures. Lap the material up the parapet walls and under the parapet caps.

Scuppers should be installed before the membrane. The membrane should go over the metal edges of the scuppers. Pay attention to sealing seams where the scuppers attach. A TPO membrane is not vapor permeable. Check with the manufacturer to see if vent stacks are recommended between the membrane and the roof sheathing.

What Your Builder Should Know

Plumbing Rough-in

What It Is

Water supply and drainpipes are installed. This is done before the cabinets and bathtubs are installed and before showers are tiled.

Categories of Concern

Mold

What Can Go Wrong Here

The bladder surrounding a shower may not be installed correctly. A bladder is a thick piece of rubber wrapped around the shower, two feet high, behind the tile. The bladder connects into the drain under the shower floor. If water leaks through a crack in the tile grout, the bladder directs it from behind the wall into the drain under the floor.

The bladder around a walk-in shower stops on each side of the walk into the shower. Water can leak into walls on each side of the entry. It's easier to waterproof

(mold-proof) the following types of showers:
- those with a step into them,
- one-piece (molded plastic) showers, or
- showers constructed with pre-made shower pans instead of custom tiled floors.

Bladder Blunders

The owner of a house complained of a mold smell. The head of their bed was against a wall opposite a walk-in shower. We cut open the wall behind the bed and found so much mold that it looked like stalagmites hanging in a cave. The entire shower needed to be gutted. The shower bladder ended on each side of the entry into the walk-in shower. It wasn't watertight.

The Alternatives

Consider not having walk-in showers. Showers with a step are easier to waterproof. Consider one-piece, molded plastic showers. They can't leak. If a shower is tiled, consider using a pre-made plastic shower pan.

Recommendations

Discuss how a shower bladder should be installed with your builder. Inspect the bladder before the shower is tiled.

Plumbing Rough-in

Request the plumber cover the floor with a tarp when cutting or gluing PVC pipe. When finished, the tarp should be carefully folded to contain the dust. Alternatively, prohibit cutting pipe inside the house. Designate a location outside and cover the ground.

Check for This

Inspect shower bladders before showers are tiled.

Ensure a leak detector is installed on the main water line.

Give This to Your Builder

Make sure shower bladders are installed correctly.

For showers with a step, install a piece of metal flashing under the tile on the step. The flashing should go down the other side, onto the shower floor, and under the tile floor, as specified in *Best Practices Guide to Residential Construction: Materials, Finishes, and Details.* The floor should be protected with a self-adhering membrane and lapped over the top of the step, similar to what is done to waterproof a flat roof.

Install an automatic shut-off to shut the water off if there is a leak. Suppliers include: WaterCop®, DIYcontrols.com, and FLO-n-STOP.™

Request plumbers cover the floor with a tarp where they cut or glue pipe or cut pipe outside in a designated location.

What Your Builder Should Know

Electrical Rough-in

What It Is

Wires are run from the fuse box to where outlets and switches will be installed.

Categories of Concern

EMFs

Shortcuts and Standard Practices

Three-way switches may be wired using the wrong type of wire. Three-way switch light switches make it possible to control a ceiling light or fixture from two locations. Three-way switches should be wired with four-wire cable. There should be a neutral, hot, ground, and *traveler* wire. The traveler wire must go to each switch. As this is cumbersome to install, an electrician may use the normal type of wire, one without a traveler, and do what is called "picking up a neutral." They connect the neutrals of the three-way switches to other lights nearby. The lights work, but the current is unbalanced on both sets of wires. If this is discovered after the house is built, the only solution, other than cutting holes in the walls and ceiling to run the correct type of wire, is to pick a switch to keep and remove the others.

What Can Go Wrong Here

You can't tell by looking at the blue prints how wires will be run over ceilings or under floors to get from the fuse box to where power is needed. It's the electrician's job to figure out how to run wires to get power where it's needed. The electrician may run wires over or under bedrooms to serve other parts of the house, something that increases EMFs in bedrooms.

The Alternatives

Think about the location of bedrooms when designing a floor plan. Design bedrooms to be at one end of the house, furthest from the main electric panel and areas that require significant amounts of power, such as the kitchen, mechanical room, water heater, and boiler.

Design for natural lighting. Specify skylights and light tubes, and have big windows.

Hard-wire the house for internet.

Install light switches near appliances to turn them off when they are not being used. These include the dishwasher and microwave oven.

Recommendations

Go over with the electrician your concern about EMFs and wiring errors. Ask them to be careful to avoid mistakes. Tell the electrician the goal is to keep wires "paired" to prevent an "unbalanced current."

To eliminate EMFs in the sleeping area, a product called a remote shut-off switch may be ordered from Safe Living Technologies. A box is installed next to the fuse box. Circuit breakers serving the bedrooms and rooms next to them are connected to the box. Inside the box, relay switches connect the circuits to the fuse box. The relay switches are opened and closed using a remote control similar to a car key. From inside the bedroom the circuit breakers can be shut off using the remote control. The effect is like camping—there is no electric field.

To minimize dirty electricity, have the electrician install light switches to shut appliances, flat panel TVs, and electronic devices that have phantom power off when they are not being used.

Hard-wire the home for internet and stereo speakers.

What Your Builder Should Know

Give This to Your Builder

26 05 00 Common Work for Electrical

When possible, avoid running wires behind or over bedrooms to serve other parts of the house.

Walls, ceilings, and floors around bedrooms should be as free as possible of wiring that serves high-current appliances, such as a water heater, freezer, boiler, stove, oven, or refrigerator.

A pool or spa pump should not be located within six feet of a bedroom or high-use room.

An insulation union (section of plastic pipe) should be inserted between metal pipes connected between the main house and a pool, well, or equipment room serviced by a separate main panel.

A dielectric union shall be installed on metallic gas and water lines where they contact an appliance, such as a water heater, boiler, or stove.

Light switches to shut the power off to the receptacle shall be installed for each of the following. The outlets shall not be split. The switch shall control the entire receptacle:

- dishwasher
- microwave oven
- potential locations for flat panel displays (TVs)

26 05 26 Grounding and Bonding

The neutral and ground busbars inside panels should be bonded only at the service entrance main disconnect (main panel). Bonding screws inside sub-panels shall be removed.

Do not bond a cable coaxial or phone ground to the electric utility ground or the metal conduit the electric company uses to mount the meter and service box.

Provide a separate grounding rod for each the phone and cable.

Electrical Rough-in

26 05 53 IDENTIFICATION FOR ELECTRICAL SYSTEMS

At the panels, all circuits will be labeled as to the area of the house and equipment served.

26 05 83 WIRING CONNECTIONS

Ensure all wiring is "paired." The following helps to prevent errors:

- All wiring in an electrical box must be of the same circuit.
- No wiring of ½ switch outlets using different breakers.
- Four-wire cable shall be used to wire three-way switches.
- 120 V appliances shall not be connected to a two-wire, 240 V service, and utilize the ground as the neutral.

27 00 00 COMMUNICATIONS

Hard-wire the home for internet using ethernet cable.
Hard-wire the house for stereo speakers.

What Your Builder Should Know

Insulation

What It Is

Insulation is installed.

Categories of Concern

VOCs
Odors

Shortcuts and Standard Practices

Few homeowners get all of the cellulose insulation they pay for. The insulation may be installed with a hose too large to pack it firm as a mattress.[1]

To prevent construction dust and debris from being inside the house for the life of the building, the house should be vacuumed before insulation and drywall are installed. This is not done.

What Can Go Wrong Here

The builder may insist on using rigid or spray foam. Spray foam off-gases and causes odors. The odors are not limited to chemicals in the foam. New odors result as foam reduces or eliminates ventilation and is exposed to heat from canned lights and heating ducts.

Rigid foams off-gas freon HFC-134a, a blowing agent used to manufacture it. A product that says "does not off-gas," means the amount is below a threshold. Freon is detected in the air in homes where it is installed.

You may have specified cellulose and didn't realize the supplier adds other ingredients. Check the Safety Data Sheet. Borax, normally added for insect and fire prevention, is non-toxic. Ammonia sulfate may be substituted, as it is cheaper. This causes ammonia odors. A manufacturer may add mineral oil. Breathing mineral oil irritates the lungs and can cause coughing and shortness of breath.

A builder may think it's a good idea to block outside air from entering the attic. The builder might stuff fiberglass insulation against the soffit vents. This causes snow to melt and water to leak inside the house where there are warm spots on the roof. The air inside an attic should be the same temperature as outside.

Insulation

The Alternatives

The common types of insulation are: fiberglass batts, blown-in fiberglass, mineral wool (rock wool) batts, blown-in cellulose, rigid foam, and spray foam. Cellulose or mineral wool is recommended. Both have high insulation values, cannot grow mold, and are good for soundproofing.

Insulation Type	Average R Value	Comment
Fiberglass batts (depending on the density)	3.1 - 5.0	
Rock wool batts	3.0 - 3.9	Higher than blown-in fiberglass
Cellulose (blown-in)	3.0 - 3.9	Same as rock wool
Fiberglass (blown-in)	2.5 - 3.7	Less than cellulose and rock wool
Polystyrene rigid foam	3.9 - 5.0	
Polyurethane and Isocyanate rigid foams	5.5 - 8.0	
Spray foams	4.0 - 8.0	

R-Value - a material's resistance to conducting heat. The higher the R-value, the more effective the insulation.

Cellulose is made with recycled newspapers and boric acid, a least toxic pest-control, flame retardant, and mold inhibitor. Rock wool (mineral wool) is made using basalt and steel slag (silicone, aluminum, magnesium, and sulfur). The mixture is heated to 3000 F and spun into fibers. The equipment may be treated with oil to keep dust down.

Cellulose may not be 100% cellulose. As the popularity of recycled products increases, manufacturers are adding jute, cotton, and 15-30% recycled polyethylene terephthalate (PET) plastic from used water and soda bottles. Mineral oil and cornstarch may be added for controlling dust.

An advantage to using mineral wool batts vs. cellulose, which is blown-in, is that batts allow for air movement. If a window leaks, and the inside of a wall has insulation blown-in, the insulation is packed too tight to allow the wall to dry. This leads to mold growing on the framing and exterior sheathing.

Choose formaldehyde-free mineral wool batts. Thermafiber® UtrlaBatt™ FF (Formaldehyde-free) mineral wool by Owens Corning is recommended.

Stone wool, mineral wool, rock wool, and slag wool are used to describe insulation made from stone or a combination of stone and steel slag. ROCKWOOL® is a trademark by Rockwool International. ROCKWOOL® reports using more rock than slag in their products compared to other brands of mineral wool. ROCKWOOL® does not have a formaldehyde-free version for framed walls. The term rock wool is henceforth used as a generic descriptor for mineral wool.

Insulation

Type of Insulation	Known Chemical Emissions	Other Possible Ingredients	Comments
Good Shepherd wool batts Breathe™batts made from hemp and flax	None	Similar to cellulose, these may have borax added as a flame retardant and for pest control.	CONSIDER Expensive
Bonded Logic UltraTouch™ (cotton) batts made from recycled blue jeans	Potential fragrance from used jeans		
Fiberglass	Formaldehyde	Resins used as binders in formaldehyde-free versions	AVOID
Rock wool batts (mineral wool)	Formaldehyde	Oil from spinning equipment and for dust control Resins used as binders in formaldehyde-free versions	CONSIDER
Cellulose (loose-fill) blown-in	Possible off-gassing from recycled newspaper content. Available with virgin paper. Some add mineral oil for dust control. Ammonia odors. Some use ammonia sulfate or magnesium sulfate for fire retardants instead of borax.	Boric acid is used as a flame retardant and for pest control. Cellulose treated with borax will not grow mold. Some add corn starch for dust control. Spray-applied may have chlorine added. Stabilized cellulose has an adhesive in the dry mix.	CONSIDER Find a brand with no additives other than borax.
Polyurethane (CFC/HCFC and pentane expanded) rigid panel foam	Isocyanates Freon	Freon (HFC-134a) is a blowing agent in polyurethane foam. Freon (HCF-142B) is a blowing agent in rigid foam.	AVOID
Polystyrene	Styrene		AVOID
Spray foam	Isocyanates and/or formaldehyde		AVOID

The resins used in formaldehyde-free fiberglass batts are acrylics and may include methyl methacrylate and butyl methacrylate[2]. These have low toxicity and may be slightly irritating to the eyes and mucus membranes. There is no published data on the emissions of resins from these batts. Odors and air quality issues have not been reported. UtrlaBatt™ by Owens Corning uses a natural, plant-based binder.

Recommendations

Cellulose or formaldehyde-free mineral wool batts are recommended.

If cellulose is used, specify a supplier who uses borax and does not add mineral oil, ammonium, or magnesium sulfate. Ask the installer to save the used bags to verify that enough insulation is being installed to achieve the desired density.

Make sure the builder does stuff insulation against soffit vents in the attic. Ask for baffles to be installed in the attic to prevent insulation blocking airflow through the soffit vents.

Insulation

Check for This

Before the insulation is installed, verify that the mechanical rough-ins are correct. If a ventilator was specified, verify the supply and return vents are installed in rooms as specified. Verify the fresh-air duct is on the side of the house, not on the roof. Verify the exhaust duct is on the roof. Check that there are pass-through registers installed in rooms that don't have return vents. These should be installed in the wall between rooms and the hallway. Make sure ducts were sealed with mastic and leak-checked.

Give This to Your Builder

The following are prohibited: spray foam, rigid foam, and fiberglass.

Blow-in cellulose or formaldehyde-free mineral wool batts shall be used for insulation.

In roofs with gables (attic spaces) baffles shall be installed to prevent insulation from blocking air flowing through the soffit vents.

07 21 23 LOOSE-FILL CELLULOSE INSULATION

The installer shall use a hose 1 1/2 to 2 inches in diameter and install a density of 3 1/2 to 4 pounds per cubic foot.

The installer shall save the used bags to check that the project is in the ballpark in terms of the density of the insulation being installed.

(1) "Dense Pack Done Right, How to Tell the Difference Between a Good Cellulose Insulation and a Bad One." Joe Riley. Fine Homebuilding. Dec 2017/Jan 2018.

(2) *Building Materials - Product Emission and Combustion Health Hazards.* Kathleen Hess-Kosa. CRC Press. 2017.

Drywall

What It Is

After the insulation is installed, drywall is hung (screwed onto the wood framing). Drywall, also known as Sheetrock® and gypsum board, comes in 4x8-foot panels. It's composed of a core of calcium sulfate (gypsum) pressed between two sheets of thick paper or fiberglass mats. Holes are cut in the drywall for electrical outlets, light fixtures, and pipes. The seams between the panels are taped with drywall tape. A white mud called joint compound is applied to create texture. The process is called "hang, tape, and mud."

In cold climates a vapor barrier is installed before the drywall is screwed to the framing. Vapor barriers are sheets of plastic that prevent moisture from breathing, cooking, and showering, from getting inside walls and roof cavities. This prevents moisture from condensing inside walls and ceilings when it's cold outside. Condensation is a source of water for mold to grow.

Categories of Concern

Mold
VOCs
Formaldehyde
Dust

Shortcuts and Standard Practices

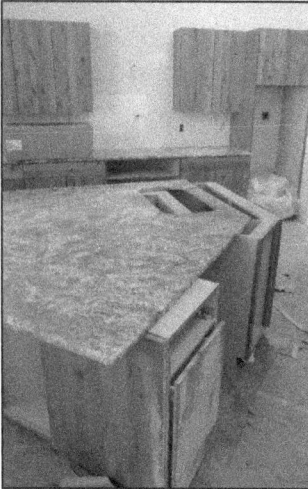

The cabinets may arrive before the drywall and painting are finished.

It's common to leave soil exposed around pipes under bathtubs. This causes mold odors. The exposed soil allows radon gas, freon in rigid foam under the slab (if used), and odors from dirt to get into the home.

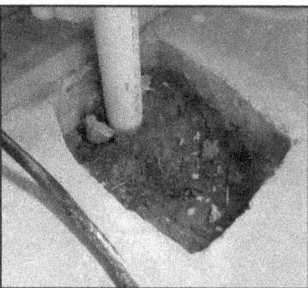

Drywall

What Can Go Wrong Here

In one house, the builder did not wait for the roof to be put on before allowing the insulation and drywall crews to start. An unexpected heavy rain caused the framing and drywall to get wet and mold to grow on walls throughout the house. It's a wonder how this happened. The building inspector is supposed to approve each step. The roof step, "dry in," should have been approved before drywall was installed.

Standard drywall has paper on both sides. Mold likes to grow on paper. Builders install "green board" in areas such as bathroom showers. Green board is paper-faced drywall treated with an antimicrobial. It will grow mold.

Drywall compound contains vinyl acetate to increase elasticity and formaldehyde and acetaldehydes as preservatives.

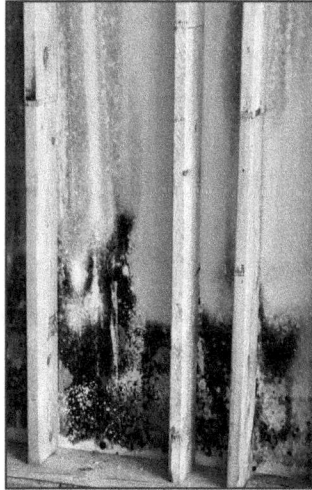

Stachybotrys mold on drywall in a house in which the drywall was installed before the roof was finished.

The Alternatives

The healthiest way is the old-fashioned method: metal lath, wood batten boards, and a cement-based plaster. This is becoming a lost art. The modern way of plastering is to install drywall and apply plaster onto the drywall. If paper-faced drywall is used, the wet plaster causes mold to grow on the drywall.

Avoid using paper-faced drywall. Use DensGlass, drywall made with fiberglass instead of paper. Fiberglass can not grow mold. Some homeowners specify it where leaks are common (around showers); others specify throughout the house and prohibit paper-faced drywall from being delivered.

Approximately thirty years ago, Georgia-Pacific invented DensGlass®. A colleague of mine in Florida was hired to test it. He set up large tanks in his office, suspended the drywall inside the tanks, and used hoses to spray the drywall and keep it wetted. No matter how he tried, he could not get mold to grow.

There are two Dens® products: DensArmor Plus® Interior Panels and DensGlass® Sheathing. DensArmor Plus® is for interior locations. DensGlass® Sheathing is used behind exterior claddings, including brick, stone, stucco, and other sidings. The term DensGlass® is used here as a generic descriptor for fiberglass-faced drywall.

Drywall

Recommendations

Make sure the roof is put on before the insulation and drywall are installed. Your builder should reschedule insulation and drywall crews until the roof is finished.

Use DensGlass® wherever drywall is required.

The main ingredient in a drywall compound (texture) should be limestone (calcium carbonate), not calcium sulfate. Consider the M-100 joint compound by Murco. It does not contain antimicrobials, formaldehyde, or vinyl acetate.

Check for This

Verify DensGlass® was used for drywall. Do not install cabinets, vanities, a water heater, or a boiler if paper-faced drywall was installed. Remove the paper-faced drywall and install DensGlass®.

Before the drywall is installed, check under bathtubs for exposed soil. Exposed soil should be sealed with concrete, mortar, or a plaster to prevent dirt and musty odors, bugs, and radon entering the home.

Give This to Your Builder

06 16 26 GYPSUM SHEATHING

DensArmor Plus® Interior Panels or DensGlass® fiberglass mat gypsum sheathing is to be used where gypsum board is required. Paper-faced gypsum board is prohibited.

06 16 53 MOISTURE-RESISTANT SHEATHING BOARD

Green board is prohibited. Use DensArmor Plus® Interior Panels or DensGlass® fiberglass mat gypsum sheathing.

09 21 16 GYPSUM BOARD ASSEMBLIES

Wall cavities shall be vacuumed and free of dust and debris before installing insulation and drywall.

Fiberglass batt insulation may not be placed inside interior wall cavities.

Drywall is to be hung with screws.

Hang drywall one-quarter inch off the floor to prevent water from wicking if there is a leak.

07 26 13 ABOVE-GRADE VAPOR RETARDERS

In cold climates a vapor barrier should be installed before installing drywall on the inside side of exterior walls and ceilings. The vapor barrier should be installed on the interior side of the framed walls and ceiling.

If cellulose is used, a vapor barrier is not required.

In humid climates, a vapor barrier should be installed on the exterior side of the framed wall.

Do not install a vapor barrier in mixed climates. Vapor barriers should never be installed on both sides of a wall. Doing so prevents drying.

Drywall

07 77 00 Air Barrier

An air barrier shall be constructed between the garage and rooms next to and above it as follows:

- Install foam sealant tape under sill plates as the walls are framed.
- After the drywall is installed, apply foam sealant tape to seal between the slab and drywall where the drywall meets the floor.
- Use spray foam to seal around penetrations for plumbing and electrical wires going into walls.
- Use sealed can lights for recessed lighting.
- Air-tighten electrical boxes by covering the back of electric boxes with the fiberglass mesh used for drywall patching and painting over the mesh with water-based duct mastic.
- After the drywall is installed, caulk around electrical boxes using silicone.
- Install gaskets on light switch plates and electrical outlets.
- The door between the house and garage should be weather-stripped.
- The doorsill and threshold should be sealed with silicone between the bottom of the threshold and slab.

22 41 19 Residential Bathtubs

Before closing the wall behind a bathtub, cover the exposed soil with concrete, mortar, or plaster.

What Your Builder Should Know

Painting

What It Is

Painting is done.

Categories of Concern

VOCs
Odors

Shortcuts and Standard Practices

A low-VOC paint may be used. Low-VOC is based on a small set of chemicals contributing to smog, not the full spectrum of possible VOCs.

Painters don't cover bare concrete or worry about dips and spills. Drips cause odors if carpet is installed over them. Large spots of paint keep glue and mortar for wood and tile floors from sticking.

What Can Go Wrong Here

A natural paint may be used. Natural paints often contain linseed oil and clay. Designers use clay paint to add color and texture. Clay will off-gas the chemicals it absorbs, like a cat box of used kitty litter. Linseed oil is a hydrocarbon and unhealthy to breathe.

Tile does not stick to drips of paint. Floor tiles become lose.

The contractor may use heaters to dry plaster or drywall texture. Heat drives moisture into walls. If it's cold outside, condensation occurs, and mold grows inside walls.

If a traditional cement-based plaster was specified, the contractor may install drywall and apply the plaster on top of the drywall. The drywall gets wet from the plaster and grows mold. This can be avoided by specifying paper-less drywall (DensGlass®).

The sealer used on plaster walls may stink.

The Alternatives

It's easy to find healthy paint. Trade brands may be healthier than natural paint. Choose paint certified GREENGUARD Gold. A paint manufacturer may choose not to pay to have a green label. The paint may have been tested and approved and listed on California's Section

Painting

1030 list. Check California's database. Look for the most expensive, healthiest paint, not just zero-VOC. Examples are Everest® by Dunn-Edwards; Natura® by Benjamin Moore; Air-Care™ by Coronado; EnviroCoat by Kelly-Moore; Harmony® by Sherwin-Williams.

Plaster should be finished and sealed using a traditional white wash after the hard-coat is dry. For a modern sealer, OKON® W-2 Water-Repellant Sealer is commonly used. It has a slight, sweet odor after it dries.

Recommendations

Choose paint certified GREENGUARD Gold or something like Everest® by Dunn-Edwards.

Make sure the painters come before flooring is installed.

Give This to Your Builder

09 91 13 EXTERIOR PAINTING

Use _____ for exterior paint.

09 92 23 INTERIOR PAINTING

Use _____ for interior paint.

Use _____ for a primer where required.

What Your Builder Should Know

Painters shall not spill or drip on concrete. Spills shall be reported, noted where they occur, and cleaned up using approved cleaning products.

09 93 13 EXTERIOR STAINING AND FINISHING

The owner shall specify acceptable and unacceptable products.

09 97 23 CONCRETE AND MASONRY COATINGS

Urethane is unacceptable.

Beeswax is unacceptable. The primary emulsifying ingredient is toluene.

Products that contain linseed are unacceptable.

Plaster shall be finished using an approved water-based sealer. Ask for samples and test spots. Products to consider include:

• MexeSeal by AFM Safecoat®
• Polyureseal BP by Safecoat®
• OKON® W-2 Water-Repellant Sealer

Note, the resin in OKON® W-2 contains acrylics and silane and siloxane. These are detected in the air in homes and may not be as low-odor as a product made by Safecoat®. OKON® W-2 may penetrate concrete and porous plaster better.

Flooring

What It Is

Wood, tile, and other types of flooring are installed.

Categories of Concern

Mold
Formaldehyde

What Can Go Wrong Here

There may be off-gassing of formaldehyde from composite (wood veneer) floors. If you test a house and find that the floor is the source of formaldehyde, the floor needs to be removed. Sealing a floor does not help.

The installer may have installed a vapor barrier under wood floors, but it was placed on top of a plywood subfloor instead of on top of the concrete. Mold can grow on the unprotected plywood.

Carpet may stink.

The Alternatives

Hardwood and ceramic tile are the healthiest types of floors. Tile is easy to clean and can not grow mold. Wood is an insulator. For those concerned about EMFs, wood insulates the body from exposure to any current that gets on the grounding system and electrifies the slab with small voltages.

Solid wood floors, finished with a healthy finish or sealer, nailed to a plywood subfloor or floated over concrete, is recommended. If there is a plywood subfloor, gluing the top flooring to the plywood may result in less formaldehyde off-gassing from the plywood.

Bamboo and cork may not be the healthiest choice. Similar to composite wood floors, the binders may contain formaldehyde or other resins that off-gas.

Recommendations

Solid wood floors or ceramic tile are recommended. Under no circumstances should composite wood flooring be installed.

For carpet, get a big piece and test it. Look for Green Label Plus, which has the strictest requirements. Roll the carpet out in the bedroom at the house you currently live in. Leave the doors and windows closed and see how long it takes for the odor to go away.

Flooring

Give This to Your Builder

Perform a calcium chloride vapor emission test before installing flooring over concrete. The manufacturer's maximum vapor emission level should be complied with.

Perform testing to make sure the pH of the slab is compatible with any adhesives that are used.

09 61 19 Concrete Floor Staining

The difficulty with a stained or painted concrete floor is finding a low-odor product that adheres. Try something certified GREENGUARD Gold.

09 64 00 Wood Flooring

Install a vapor barrier under wood in contact with concrete. The vapor barrier should be placed in direct contact with the slab.

Do not install wood floors below grade.

Wood should be finished off-site and allowed to dry before being brought inside.

Allow wood to acclimatize before installing it by letting the finished wood sit in the room it will be installed in for thirty days. This prevents swelling and shrinking from changes in moisture content after it is installed.

If wood will be glued to a concrete floor, cover the floor with drop cloths when the walls are painted. The glue will act as the vapor barrier. Glue won't stick to paint. Ensure there is good coverage.

09 68 00 Carpeting

Do not glue carpet. Use nail tack strips and seam tape.

What Your Builder Should Know

Doors, Cabinets, and Trim

What It Is

The interior doors are hung, cabinets are installed, and baseboards, trim, and moldings are put on. Wood floors may be sanded and have a first finish coat applied.

Categories of Concern

Formaldehyde
Drywall dust
Wood dust

What Can Go Wrong Here

Assumptions may have been made about how much formaldehyde kitchen cabinets emit. Once installed, there may be an odor, exacerbated if a ventilation system is not installed. The only solution will be to remove the cabinets.

The Alternatives

Use real wood. If cabinets cannot be constructed with solid-dimensional, real wood, consider not having cabinet doors—have solid wood shelves and glass doors.

An option is to use solid wood for doors and drawer faces and formaldehyde-free sheet goods for the remainder of the cabinet. This will not mean there is no odor. Some of the resins substituted for formaldehyde glues have an odor.

Low-formaldehyde sheet goods include the following:

- Medex® and Medite®II by Roseburg. MDF (medium density fiberboard).

- SkyBlend® by Roseburg. Particleboard made with recycled wood fibers and an ultra low emitting formaldehyde resin (ULEF).

- TemStock® by Georgia-Pacific. Particleboard made from recycled wood with no added formaldehyde resins.

Specify Elmer's® Carpenter's Wood Glue and the acceptable stains, primers, and finishes. Finishes should be applied off-site.

Doors, Cabinets, and Trim

If you don't want to custom build the cabinets, sources of pre-made cabinets to consider include:

• Core Cabinets & Design, Inc.

• Neil Kelly

Metal cabinets have the benefit of being chemical free, but they conduct, acting as an antenna for EMFs.

Recommendations

Request the builder not allow cabinets to be delivered until the drywall is installed and painted. If cabinets arrive early, they should be sealed with plastic and stored in a dry, clean location.

What Your Builder Should Know

Countertops

What It Is

Countertops are installed.

Categories of Concern

Formaldehyde
VOCs
EMFs

What Can Go Wrong Here

Laminate counter tops are normally applied over particleboard or plywood that contain formaldehyde. There may be high levels of VOCs from the resins used in formaldehyde-free products.

The Alternatives

Solid surface countertops are recommended and include the following:

- Granite. A hot spot of radioactivity the size of a dime is normal and not a health hazard.

- Natural and composite quartz materials. These have an advantage over granite in that they don't need to be sealed. Brands include: Cambria®, Silestone®, Zodiaq®, Caesarstone®, and EuroStone®.

- Corain®, Avonite®, Swanstone®, PaperStone®

Recommendations

Tell your builder what you decide.

Tile

What It Is

Tile floors and shower tile are installed.

Categories of Concern

VOCs
Mold

What Can Go Wrong Here

There may be a wood-framed, tiled seat in a shower. When someone sits on it, the wood framing flexes and the grout cracks, allowing water to seep into walls around the shower and under the seat.

An odor may persist if a petroleum-based grout sealer is used.

Recommendations

Install wood benches (open underneath the bench) in showers. If there is tiled seat, fill the inside with concrete to prevent the seat from flexing when someone sits on it.

Use a water-based grout sealer.

Give This to Your Builder

GROUT SEALERS

Grout should be clean and dry before applying a sealer.

Sealers containing petroleum and solvents are prohibited.

The following are acceptable. Test a small area for adhesion and curing before applying to the entire shower:

- AFM Safecoat® Grout Sealer
- AFM Safecoat® Safe Seal. It may be diluted with water 50:50 and mixed into dry grout.
- Sodium silicate (water glass), a clear sealer painted over grout.

Appliances

What It Is

After the cabinets are installed and the flooring is finished, appliances are installed. These include the stove, refrigerator, dishwasher, washer, and dryer.

Categories of Concern

Natural gas and propane leaks
EMFs

Shortcuts and Standard Practices

Appliance service technicians don't have meters to check for gas leaks and carbon monoxide. Contractors may use soapsuds. Suds and bubbles will not identify small gas leaks. If carbon monoxide is measured, the contractor may turn the meter on in the middle of the room. To accurately test gas appliances for safety, a probe must be inserted into the exhaust.

What Can Go Wrong Here

Natural gas and propane are known to induce or worsen allergy and asthma. Burning gas creates nitrogen oxide, known to cause asthma. Gas may be a factor in Sudden Infant Death Syndrome (SIDS).

Because the combustion efficiency is 100%, a manufacturer may say a gas fireplace doesn't need to be vented. The main by-product of combustion is water vapor. Excessive vapor leads to condensation and mold.

There may be a high magnetic field near an appliance, even if it is off. This is because the digital displays, clocks, and circuits are always on.

The Alternatives

Consider going all electric. At a minimum, have an electric oven and an electric range.

If you have gas, install a big hood with a wide girth over the stove. There cannot be a microwave above a range, as it would be in the way of the exhaust duct.

Suggestions of testing appliances for gas leaks and carbon monoxide are in the chapter for doing a final walk-through with the builder.

Appliances

Recommendations

Electric, on-demand water heaters are recommended. These save money on heating bills, provide endless hot water, and require little space.

If you have a gas water heater or boiler, it should be the sealed-combustion type and power-vented outside.

Give This to Your Builder

22 33 00 FUEL-FIRED WATER HEATERS

Gas water heaters shall be on-demand and sealed combustion, power-vented outside.

22 33 30 ELECTRIC WATER HEATERS

Water heaters shall be on-demand.

23 51 13 CHIMNEYS - DRAFT-INDUCTION FANS

A draft inducer fan should be installed on top of chimneys to overcome the effects of wind, cold surfaces, and downdrafts.

What Your Builder Should Know

Plumbing Finish Work

What It Is

The plumber comes back to put in toilets, sinks, faucets, and fixtures. This is called trimming-out.

Categories of Concern

Water leaks and flooding
Odors
Mold

What Can Go Wrong Here

The floor plan may not allow room for installing the water treatment tanks required for a whole-house system to remove chlorine.

Leaks may occur when the water is turned on. Without an automatic shut-off, the builder may return the next day to flooding.

The Alternatives

Before breaking ground, obtain a copy of the city water report or test the well water. Determine what kinds of filters are required and design for a place to put the treatment tanks and filters in the house.

Recommendations

For well water, install a UV disinfection system on the line coming from the well.

For city water, specify a whole-house carbon tank to remove chlorine.

Install a reverse osmosis (RO) filter under the kitchen sink for drinking water. Efficiencies are as high as 98% for most contaminants.

Additional treatments may be required depending on what is in the water. Be cautious about all-in-one treatment systems. Hard water makes them less effective.

Understand how a shower bladder should be installed. Ask the installer to provide a detailed drawing of how it will be installed.

To minimize the amount of mold that can grow if drywall gets wet, ensure DensGlass® is installed on both sides of walls around showers. For example, the builder may use cement backer board to install the shower tile around the showers. That's fine. The walls on the other side of the shower (bedrooms, hallway, and so forth) need to be constructed with DensGlass®.

Give This to Your Builder

22 31 00 WATER SOFTENERS

Install a water softener to treat hard water.

22 32 00 WATER FILTRATION EQUIPMENT

For city water, a whole-house tank carbon filter should be installed to remove chlorine as it enters the house.

A reverse osmosis (RO) filter should be installed under the kitchen sink.

Install a UV (ultraviolet light) disinfection system on a line coming from a well.

Install other water filtration equipment as needed based on the water quality testing report and the owners' specifications.

22 51 19 SWIMMING POOL WATER TREATMENT EQUIPMENT AND HOT TUBS

Install a non-chlorine sanitizer for pool and hot tub sanitation. Bromine is toxic. A copper and silver treatment system is recommended such as those manufactured by Lifeguard Purification Systems (813) 875-7777.

Maintain the proper pool water chemistry (pH and hardness).

Use a non-chlorine product such as potassium permanganate for shock treatment as required.

22 41 16 RESIDENTIAL SINKS

Caulk the backs of vanities and behind sink back-splashes to prevent water dripping behind vanities.

Electrical Finish Work

What It Is

The electrician comes back to connect outlets, light fixtures, switches, ceiling fans, and so forth. The furnace and air-conditioner will be connected.

Categories of Concern

EMFs
Mercury

What Can Go Wrong Here

Florescent and compact florescent light bulbs (CFL), light-emitting diode (LED) bulbs, and similar energy-saving light bulbs cause headache and fatigue and impair concentration. When these bulbs are used, current ends up on the grounding system, and an EMF called dirty electricity (harmonically distorted voltage) is created.

CFL and florescent light bulbs contain mercury. If one of these bulbs breaks in the house, the house is contaminated with mercury.

What Your Builder Should Know

Cable and phone companies connect their ground wires to the ground used by the electric company. This allows current to get on the ground of the wires inside the house and creates a magnetic field.

As soon as you plug something in—a lamp or light fixture—the unshielded cord brings the electric field out into the open. In bedrooms, living rooms, and where a lot of time is spent, replace the cords on lamps and light fixtures with shielded cords.

The Alternatives

Do not have energy saving light bulbs. Old-fashioned, incandescent light bulbs are the best for creating a healthy environment and reducing stress. These are no longer available in high-wattage bulbs. As needed, use several low-watt incandescent bulbs.

Low-voltage, decorative lighting requires a transformer. Transformers create magnetic fields. If you have low-voltage lighting, do not place the transformer on the ceiling under a bedroom.

Consider using outdoor halogen spotlights for interior canned lights. Halogens resemble natural light and, unlike LEDs, don't contain an electronic ballast.

Electrical Finish Work

Give This to Your Builder

26 09 33 CENTRAL DIMMING CONTROLS

Dimmer switches are prohibited.

26 22 00 LOW-VOLTAGE TRANSFORMERS

Transformers for low-voltage lighting shall not be installed on the ceiling below a bedroom.

26 50 00 LIGHTING

There shall not be any of the following:

- fluorescent light bulbs
- CFL light bulbs
- LED light bulbs
- low-voltage lighting that requires a transformer
- dimmer switches

The cords on light fixtures shall be retrofitted with shielded cable. Belden makes the recommended cable. Use 14/2 for 15 amps, 18/2 for 10 amps. The 18/2 is thinner and easier to retrofit into light fixtures.

What Your Builder Should Know

HVAC Finish Work

What It Is

The HVAC contractor comes back to install duct registers and get the furnace and air conditioner running.

Categories of Concern

Ventilation
VOCs

What Can Go Wrong Here

You didn't pick the best HEPA filter for the furnace or air-conditioner.

You didn't specify a ventilator, or the builder's idea of ventilation is different than yours.

No Means No

Edward and his wife were considering buying a spec

house. They picked a lot, chose a floor plan, and purchased the yet-to-be-built house. They understood that
the builder did not install ventilators in the homes being
built. Edward asked if he could have a ventilator installed
if he paid extra for one. The builder said no. Edward
asked if he could have someone else install a ventilator
before the builder finished the house. The answer was
no. The home would need to be retrofitted with a ventilator after the house was finished. This meant cutting
into drywall and installing ducts after it was finished.

Recommendations

Discuss with your builder specifications for installing the
ventilator and the ductwork when you first meet.

Final Finish Work

What It Is

Accessories are installed. These include window, door, and closet hardware, window screens, shower doors, and mirrors. Paint touch-ups and drywall repairs are done. The last finish on a wood floor may be done. Carpet is installed as heavy foot traffic is over.

Categories of Concern

Formaldehyde
VOCs

Shortcuts and Standard Practices

It's standard to use particleboard to build shelves in walk-in closets and kitchen pantries. Using low-formaldehyde wood may result in high levels of formaldehyde, depending on how much wood is installed and the amount of ventilation.

What Can Go Wrong Here

Carpet may stink. Vinyl and nylon window and door screens may stink. Standard hollow interior doors may off-gas formaldehyde from particleboard and MDF board.

The Alternatives

Shelving

Use solid wood to build cabinets and shelves in walk-in closets and pantries.

Doors

Consider solid wood doors. If using stock manufactured doors, seal the doors to prevent off-gassing using a Safecoat® product. Seal all six sides before the doors are installed.

Screens

Aluminum screens off-gas less than vinyl, nylon, and fiberglass.

Flooring

Ceramic tile or solid, hardwood floors are healthier than carpet. For example, 3/4-inch hardwood Oak, nailed instead of glued. Make sure a vapor barrier is installed under wood in contact with concrete. The vapor barrier should go on top of the concrete.

Concrete

For stained or painted concrete, consider products certified by GREENGUARD Gold. Test products for adhesion and odors on scraps of concrete. Apply the product to a piece of concrete and let it dry. Place the dry sample in a glass jar in the sun for a day. Crack the lid and check if there is an odor. If there is an odor find a different product.

Carpet

The healthiest carpet is made of untreated wool without insecticides or mothproofing. High-quality rugs with natural fibers are a substitute for carpet. Be cautious choosing carpet based on labels. The Green Label Program tests for only thirteen chemicals and calculates permissible emission levels based on a commercial building ventilated with fresh outdoor air. Avoid bonded urethane (rebond), the multi-colored, foam carpet pad. The glue that bonds the colored scraps of foam together contains formaldehyde.

What Your Builder Should Know

Recommendations

Under no circumstances should particleboard be used.
Use real, solid-dimensional wood to build cabinets and
shelves in walk-in closets.

Give This to Your Builder

Solid dimensional, real wood must be used for applications such as
shelving in walk-in and built-in closets. If composite wood
materials are required, use ultra low emission formaldehyde
(ULEF) or no added formaldehyde (NAF) wood.

Wood floors should be finished off-site and dry before being
brought into the home. Allow the finished wood to acclimatize by
storing it in the room it will be installed in for thirty days. This
prevents swelling and shrinking if the wood's moisture content
changes after it is installed.

When the windows and doors arrive, remove the screens and air
them out.

A calcium chloride vapor-emission test should be performed
before installing ceramic tile. Wait until the test indicates the level
of vapor emitted from the slab is lower than the maximum the
manufacturer recommends. Mortar shall not be allowed to sit idle.

Cleaning Up

What It Is

A final cleaning is done.

Categories of Concern

Dust

What Can Go Wrong Here

The floors look clean; dust is hidden under and on top of cabinets, on top of and under appliances, inside walls, and in furnace ducts.

Recommendations

Request that the builder clean the house at the end of each day.

Request that the builder keep the air ducts sealed and not use them during construction.

Have the insides of wall cavities vacuumed before the insulation is installed.

If the house is really dusty consider cleaning the house following the protocol in the Appendix. This is more applicable to houses with wood and tile floors, and not carpet, as the carpet will get dirty. It may work if the carpet is first protected with a non-slip covering.

Give This to Your Builder

01 74 16 Site Maintenance

The site, including sidewalks, driveways, parking areas, building entrances, and the street, shall be kept clean and free of debris. These shall be cleaned daily.

At the end of each day, construction and personal waste shall be removed from the interior of the home, including the garage. Waste bins used to collect scraps of wood, drywall, pipe, and so forth, shall be emptied. The floors shall be vacuumed, including the garage.

01 74 23 Final Cleaning

Prior to the walk-through, a final cleaning shall be performed using the approved methods and cleaning products.

The Final Walk-through

What It Is

This is the final walk-through with the builder. All the systems should have been commissioned, during which testing was performed to verify that the mechanical and ventilation systems are working. It doesn't mean they are working as specified.

Shortcuts and Standard Practices

The final walk-through is a dog and pony show. The focus is on how nice the house looks. Unless you give the builder the following specs, you may not realize a problem until you move in.

What Can Go Wrong Here

In a study of 46 new homes, homeowners were polled if they were knowledgeable about the ventilation system in their homes. 50% said they were. When researchers went to the homes, they found the ventilators to be working in only one home.

Recommendations

Hire a general home inspector to go with you and to perform a pre-purchase home inspection.

Ask the contractor to verify the ventilation system works as designed.

If you are lucky, it will rain. Check under the corners of windows using a moisture meter. If elevated moisture readings are observed, the cause is the windows were not flashed correctly. The only way to fix the problem is to remove the windows and re-install them with the flashing done correctly.

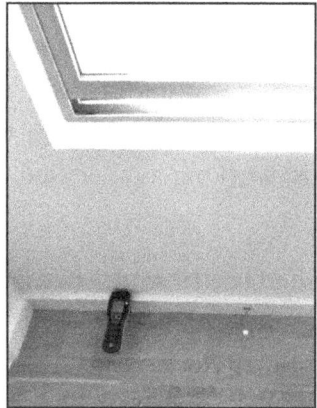

Use the pins on a moisture meter to check for leaks under windows.

If it's a green building, a Residential Energy Services Network (RESNET) professional will have tested how leaky the ducts are. Duct leakage is reported as duct leakage @ 25 pascals, the pressure the system is at when the furnace or air-conditioning is running. The International Energy Conservation Code (IECC) allows a maximum of 3 to 4 CFMs of leakage for every 100 square feet of house. Factoring in the square feet of a house allows larger homes to have higher leakages as they have more ducts. For example, if the paperwork says the duct leakage is 80 CMF, a home must be at least 2,000 square feet for that to be acceptable.

Give This to Your Builder

01 70 00 Execution & Closeout Requirements

01 75 13.01 Check Gas Fittings for Leaks

Gas pipefittings and flex hoses shall be checked for gas leaks using a combustible gas sniffer. Flex hoses that leak shall be replaced, not tightened.

01 75 13.02 Adjust and Replace Orifices on Gas Ovens

Carbon monoxide should be measured at the stovetop and inside ovens. The orifice for an oven should be adjusted or replaced with a smaller one as necessary to reduce the amount of carbon monoxide produced to less than 100 ppm. For levels above 100 ppm, the stove/oven shall be replaced.

01 75 13.03 Measure Carbon Monoxide

A professional shall measure carbon monoxide at each gas appliance. A probe shall be inserted into the flue or exhaust. If a level of greater than 100 ppm is measured, the appliance shall be repaired or replaced.

01 75 13.10 Check the Ventilation System

Verify the fresh-air ventilator (ERV or HRV) is operating as specified.

01 75 13.15 Check the Make-up air for the Dryer

Turn the dryer on and verify that the fresh-air intake for the outdoor make-up air vent opens. Using a manometer, verify that a negative air pressure is not created in the home when the dryer is running.

01 75 13.12 Check the Garage Exhaust Fan

Verify that the exhaust fan in the garage works. It should be configured to run continuously and have the switch labeled to leave it on.

01 75 13.16 Check the Make-up air for Kitchen Range Hood

Turn the kitchen range hood on and verify that the fresh-air intake vent to the kitchen opens. Use a manometer to verify that a negative air pressure is not created in the kitchen when the range hood is on.

01 75 13.20 Inspect the HVAC System

Inspect the inside of the HVAC system. Check there is no exposed fiberglass or black felt material visible inside the blower compartment. These should be covered with foil and secured with foil tape.

Check the HVAC system and ducts are clean and were not used during construction. If the system is dirty or was used, have it cleaned by a professional. Sanitizers and antimicrobial products are prohibited. A duct cleaning company should stick to physical cleaning methods—air hoses, air whips, and brushes. If the ducts have visible debris inside them they should be replaced.

01 75 13.25 VERIFY THE CONDENSATE PAN DRAINS

Cycle the air-conditioner and verify that water collects in the pan and drains properly. When finished with the HVAC inspection, seal the access panels with foil tape.

01 81 19.10 ELECTROMAGNETIC FIELD TESTING

Turn on all the lights. Leave them on and walk through the house with a gauss meter. Watch the meter as someone turns on and off each light. If the readings change, the electrician used the wrong type of wire to install the three-way switches or there is another error causing the current to be unbalanced on a set of wires. For information on how to locate and repair wiring errors that cause elevated magnetic fields, see the book *Unplugged: How to Find and Get Rid of EMFs in Your Home.*

01 81 19.20 TESTING FOR MOLD

If a roof or plumbing leak occurred during construction, or staining is visible on a wall or a ceiling, an assessment for mold should be performed by a Certified Microbial Consultant (CMC), board-awarded by the American Council for Certification (ACAC). Go to the website acac.org and enter your zip code to find a consultant.

01 81 19 INDOOR AIR QUALITY REQUIREMENTS

A short-term test for radon shall be performed with the radon mitigation system turned off. If the test results indicate the level is high (greater than 4.0 piC/l), turn the system on and re-test the home 24 hours later. If the short-term test shows the level is within EPA limits, leave the system off and start a long-term ninety-day test. The long-term test may be performed under normal conditions, with doors and windows open or closed as they normally would be.

01 1 91 COMMISSIONING

Provide the homeowner with an operations and maintenance manual for the mechanical and electrical systems.

Driveways and Landscaping

What It Is

Once the heavy trucks and equipment are gone, the driveway and walkways may be finished. A landscaper may plant grass, shrubs, trees, make flowerbeds, mulch, and do other work.

Categories of Concern

Mold
Odors

Shortcuts and Standard Practices

Landscapers push dirt up against the finished house. This can cause problems related to mold. The dirt may block the weep holes at the bottom of siding. Unless the slab was poured with more than four inches of clearance between it and the ground, when landscaping is finished the ground may be at the same level as the floor inside the house. Water can leak inside.

What Can Go Wrong Here

Asphalt is made with crude oil. Although fumes may dissipate after the asphalt is dry, there may be odors on hot days.

The Alternatives

Use brick pavers or concrete for driveways.

Give This to Your Builder

Dirt, rocks, lawn, and other landscaping must not be next to the house higher than what is required to maintain at four inches of clearance between the bottom of siding and soft grade (landscaping) and two inches of clearance between the bottom of siding and hard grade (sidewalks, driveways, patios).

Landscape should slope away from the foundation. Water should drain away from the house around the perimeter.

Checking the Builder's Work

These are the key elements to check during construction. It may be helpful to hire a general home inspector to go with you to answer questions and provide an opinion independent from your builder's.

BEFORE THE SLAB IS POURED

Inspect the vapor barrier. Make sure there is one and that it is placed on top of gravel, not sand. Make sure it's watertight. The sealant tape sold with the vapor barrier material should have been used to seal around plumbing pipes and electrical conduits that penetrate the slab. Make sure a radon mitigation system (pipes are placed in the gravel with risers where the radon mitigation consultant specified them) is installed.

AFTER THE SLAB IS POURED

Check for cracks in the concrete. Cracks and control

joints should be sealed with silicone caulk. Seal around pipes and electrical conduits where they penetrate the slab. Check there is four inches of clearance between the top of the slab and the ground.

WHEN WOOD ARRIVES

Verify that the wood delivered is clean and free of mold. Check the wood with the pins of a moisture meter. Do not accept wood with moisture readings greater than 19%. Make sure the builder has designated a place to store wood where it will be covered and protected from rain and snow. Check to see that the builder has a copy of the moisture management plan and has informed everyone on the project there is one.

AFTER FRAMING IS COMPLETED, BEFORE PLYWOOD OR OSB SHEATHING IS INSTALLED ON THE OUTSIDE WALLS

Inspect the wood framing for mold. If mold is present, stop work and consult a mold inspector for remediation. The simplest method of removing mold (other than removing the wood) is blasting with dry ice. A light blasting is sufficient. The used dry ice pellets evaporate. Sandblasting is not ideal because of the amount of silica dust created. Alternatively, hand sanding with a power sander and wire brush is preferred. Afterwards a leaf blower should be used to blow the dust off the wood and out of the house.

AFTER THE HOUSEWRAP IS INSTALLED, BEFORE ANY WINDOWS ARE INSTALLED

Inspect the housewrap for tears. Tears shall be mended using housewrap tape.

AFTER THE FIRST WINDOW IS INSTALLED

Ask the builder to have one window flashed and allow you to inspect it before the rest of the windows are flashed. Windows should not be flashed until all of the sheathing, housewrap, and building paper are installed on the house. If a window is flashed correctly, the bottom flange and nails should be visible. Imagine you are a drop of rainwater. Starting from the top of the wall where it meets the roof, imagine dripping down. Is there a way you can get inside? Can you find a way in on the top, sides, or bottom of the window? If so, there is a better way to flash the windows.

AFTER THE SIDING IS INSTALLED

Siding should terminate at the top of the slab and not continue past it to the ground.

Check there is a minimum of two inches between the bottom of the siding and hard surfaces (driveways, porches, sidewalks) and four inches between the bottom of the siding and soft grade (landscaping, dirt). For stucco, make sure a weep screed is installed at the bottom of the stucco and that the weep holes are not covered by stucco or paint.

AFTER THE ROOF UNDERLAYMENT (BUILDING PAPER) IS INSTALLED, **BEFORE** THE REMAINDER OF THE ROOFING MATERIALS ARE INSTALLED

Ask a roofer or home inspector who has expert knowledgeable about flashing to go with you. Check the proper flashing is installed around and next to chimneys, dormers, valleys (sections of roofs meeting), skylights, sidewalls (where the roof touches a wall on the side of the house), above doors, and above windows.

BEFORE SHOWER TILE IS INSTALLED

Inspect the shower bladders. Make sure they are water tight and connected to the drain under the shower floor.

BEFORE INSULATION IS INSTALLED

Verify the interior of the walls have been vacuumed and are clean of construction debris. If they are not vacuumed, you will have sawdust and debris inside the walls for the life of the building.

Verify the ductwork for the ventilator is installed. Check for supply and return vents in the rooms you requested them. If there are supposed to be pass-through vents installed in rooms without return ducts, verify those are installed. Verify the fresh-air intake is located on the side of the house, not the roof. Verify the exhaust duct is on the roof. Make sure the ducts were sealed with mastic and leak-checked.

Before drywall is installed

Check under bathtubs for exposed soil. Exposed soil should be covered with concrete, mortar, or plaster.

Before installing cabinets, vanities, and appliances

Verify DensGlass® is installed in locations that might get wet: behind and next to kitchen and bathroom sink cabinets, around inside the perimeter of the water heater closet, behind the dishwasher, behind the washing machine, in rooms next to and opposite showers, and so forth. If you prohibited paper-faced drywall from being used, this should not be an issue.

The Top 10 Lists

Top 10 Things to Do to Prevent Mold

1. Wear big boots. Build on a concrete slab with a minimum of four inches between the bottom of the siding and the ground. Do not have a basement or crawlspace.

2. Avoid housewrap. Install two layers of traditional Grade D building paper. If code requires housewrap, put the housewrap on first, and cover it with a layer of building paper.

3. Flash the windows the correct way.

4. Inspect wood as it arrives for mold and dampness. Measure wood with a moisture meter. Readings should be 19% or less. If the readings are greater than 19% or the wood looks as if it might have mold, don't accept the wood. Store wood to keep it dry.

5. Discuss with your builder how to design and build showers. Inspect shower bladders as they are installed.

6. Install an automatic shut-off that shuts the water main off if there is a plumbing leak.

7. Wear a big hat. A well constructed, pitched roof, should include flashing around doors and windows, side-walls, chimneys, and skylights.

8. Ventilate it. Install an ERV or HRV and a system of ductwork dedicated to the ventilation system.

9. Build a test structure and have the contractor leak test it. Leak test the house before the siding goes on. Spray around doors and over windows. If the builder worries about water leaking in, it's not a good idea to put the siding on until it's weatherproofed adequately.

10. Maintain the house. Twice a year, get on a ladder and caulk the tops and sides of windows, and penetrations around light fixtures, outlets, and so forth.

Top 10 Things to Do to Reduce EMFs

1. Measure the level of the magnetic field at the site before building. Do not buy or build on a lot with high fields.

2. Avoid metal framing.

3. Don't put rebar in or under the concrete. Rebar in the footer is acceptable. Rebar in the slab is not.

4. Avoid romex, the normal type of wiring used to wire a home. Use health care facility (HCF) or electrical metallic tubing (EMT) for wiring.

5. Think about the floor plan. Put the fuse box far from locations you spend time in and away from bedrooms and living rooms. The best place for bedrooms is at the end of a house, on a corner. Do not put a bed against a wall where an electrical appliance such as a refrigerator or water heater is on the other side.

6. Do not have florescent or energy-saving light bulbs.

7. Do not install dimmer switches.

8. Wire the house for internet and stereo to limit the use of WiFi and bluetooth. (Bluetooth® is a registered trademark and used here as a generic descriptor similar to coke, xerox, and kleenex.)

9. Talk to the electrician about how to avoid the common types of mistakes that result in net current and magnetic fields. Tell the electrician to keep all the wires "paired" to keep the current "balanced."

10. Install kill switches (light switches) for appliances (dishwasher, microwave, washer, dryer) to shut them off when they are not used.

Top 10 Things to Do for Good Air (Low VOCs)

1. Pick a healthy location. Do not build near a highway or business such as a dry cleaner or auto shop. Pick a lot at the end of a one-way street, in a cul-de-sac, with no drive-by traffic.

2. Build on a concrete slab. Do not have a basement or crawlspace.

3. Avoid housewrap. Use two layers of traditional building paper instead.

4. Use cellulose or mineral wool batts for insulation. Avoid spray and rigid foams.

5. Use real wood for cabinets and built-in shelves in walk-in closets and pantries.

6. Minimize carpet. Solid wood (not composite wood) and ceramic tile are the healthiest types of floors.

7. Ventilate the house with outdoor air. Install an ERV or HRV ventilator with ductwork dedicated to the ventilator. Don't use bathroom fans or the kitchen range to ventilate the house. Ventilators should not share ductwork with the furnace or air-conditioner or be connected to the bathroom or kitchen fans.

8. Connect a good HEPA filter to the furnace or air-conditioner. A Pure Air Systems 600HS Plus is recommended.

9. Install an exhaust fan on the ceiling in the garage. Run it all of the time.

10. Go all-electric. Do not have natural gas or propane.

The Big Top 10

This combines the most important elements for preventing mold, reducing EMFs, and creating healthy indoor air.

1. Ventilate it. Install a ventilator to ventilate the house with fresh outdoor air. The ventilator should have its own ductwork. The bathroom fans or kitchen range hood should not be used for ventilation. Those should be dedicated to source control. Install an exhaust fan in the garage and keep it on all the time.

2. Go all-electric. Avoid gas and propane.

3. Do not use romex wiring. Use health care facility (HCF) or electrical metallic tubing (EMT) for wiring.

4. Use real wood for kitchen cabinets and to build storage cabinets and shelves in walk-in closets.

5. Use blown-in cellulose or mineral wool batts for insu-

lation.

6. Build on a concrete slab. Do not have a basement or crawlspace.

7. Use DensGlass®, drywall that has fiberglass on the outside instead of paper, wherever drywall is required.

8. Make sure the windows are flashed the correct way. Use a peel-and-stick membrane three inches wider than the width of the framing. Watch the builder flash and install the first window to make sure it's done right.

9. Do not have florescent or compact (CFL) light bulbs.

10. In older houses, test materials for asbestos and lead-based paint before they are removed or disturbed.

Specifications by Category

I've been told builders do not like to read. The following are abbreviated versions of the specifications found at the end of each chapter.

Specifications for Preventing Mold

Drywall

Paper-faced drywall is prohibited. If paper-faced drywall is delivered, it should be refused. DensGlass® shall be used anywhere drywall, including green board, would normally be used. Screws shall be used to install the drywall. Hang drywall one-quarter inch off the floor to prevent water from wicking if there is a leak.

Moisture Management Plan

A moisture management plan shall be kept on-site for all to reference as follows:

Contact the lumber company and tell them we will not accept moldy wood.

When lumber arrives, it shall be tested with the pins on a moisture meter. If it reads greater than 19% moisture, the lumber shall be refused for delivery.

What Your Builder Should Know

Wood should be stored on palettes, cross-stacked, and covered with a tarp to protect it from rain and snow. Do not cover airtight. Allow for ventilation.

If it rains after the house is framed, wood shall be tested with a moisture meter. If it is greater than 19% for more than two days, work shall stop. The house framing shall not be closed until the wood has dried to less than or equal to 19% moisture readings and is inspected for mold.

Air Barrier

Building paper shall be used instead of housewrap. If code requires housewrap, install a layer of building paper on top of the housewrap. An inspection of the house-wrap for tears, and repairs shall be made before installing the building paper. Tears shall be mended using house-wrap tape.

Leak Detectors

Install an automatic leak detector at the main shut-off.

Shower Bladders

The installation of shower bladders shall be done according to *Best Practices Guide to Residential Construction: Materials, Finishes, and Details.*

Specifications for Preventing Mold

Water Should Drain Away From the House

Back-fill and compact soil as necessary to raise the level of the foundation such that the finished slab will be a minimum of four inches above the ground and finished landscaping.

Gas Generators and Gas Heaters

Gas generators and gas heaters are prohibited in the house and garage. Electric heaters, powered by a gas generator, outside and away from the house, are acceptable.

Install a Vapor Retarder (Barrier) Under the Slab

Six to eight inches of clean, dry, one-half-inch gravel shall be installed under the vapor barrier. Overlap the seams six inches and seal them with the sealant tape supplied by the manufacturer. Lap the vapor barrier over the footing and seal it to the foundation. Seal around electrical conduits and pipes penetrating the slab using the sealant tape provided by the manufacturer of the vapor barrier material. The vapor barrier shall be watertight. Tears and punctures should be repaired with the sealant tape.

In Humid Climates

Install a UV light to shine directly on the HVAC coils.

What Your Builder Should Know

Install an Aprilaire® Ultra-Aire Whole House Dehumidifier or similar type system to aid with dehumidification.

In Cold Climates

Install a self-adhering underlayment, such as Ice & Water Shield®, on the roof.

Ensure the Correct Flashing is Installed

This includes primary and secondary (roof return) kick-out flashing, step flashing, chimney cap flashing, saddles, crickets, and around skylights.

Exterior Doors

When the doors arrive, remove the metal pieces on the bottom and caulk between the bottom piece and door.

A metal pan flashing should be installed under the thresholds of exterior doors. The pan should slope from the grade of the finished flooring, under the door, and lap down the outside of the foundation.

The top and sides of framing around exterior doors should be flashed before the doors are hung.

Flash the Windows the Correct Way

Do not install the windows or window flashing until all

Specifications for Preventing Mold

of the sheathing and building paper and/or housewrap are installed. The flashing membrane needs to be the depth of the sill plus a few extra inches to lap down the exterior wall, over the housewrap or building paper. For example, if the framing is 2 x 6 construction, a flashing membrane of nine inches is required.

For RECESSED windows, the entire window opening and framing around the windows should be flashed before the window is inserted.

For windows FLAT with the exterior sheathing, flash the windows as follows:

1. Cut a hole in the building paper and/or housewrap and fold it back.

2. Place a sill pan on the windowsill. Manufactured pan flashing systems include the Weathermate™Sill Pan by Dow®.

3. Install peel-and-stick flashing over the pan and up the framing on each side of the window to the top of the window. The flashing should extend over the front edge of the windowsill and overlap the framing and building paper on the bottom and sides of the window three inches.

4. Before inserting the window, caulk behind the top and side flanges of the window, taking care to cover the nail holes. Do not caulk the bottom flange. Water needs to

escape out the bottom.

5. Insert the window.

6. Nail or screw the window in place. Do not spray foam between the framing and windows for insulation or to make them airtight. Foam is not waterproof and interferes with drainage.

7. Install peel-and-stick flashing on each side of the window, extending a few inches above and below the window. The peel-and-stick should go over the building paper.

8. Use a roller to press the flashing tight against the building to ensure a good bond.

9. Apply peel and stick flashing across the top of the window, lapping it across the peel-and-sticks applied on the sides.

10. Pull the housewrap and building paper down over the top of the window.

Flashing should not be installed on the bottom of the window after the window is inserted. Water needs to be able to drip out the bottom of the window, onto the flashing, and onto the building paper outside the house. Do not caulk the bottom of the window. Caulk is not required and interferes with water draining from the bottom of the window onto the flashing and building paper.

Specifications for Reducing EMFs

Wiring Materials

Romex is prohibited. Wiring shall be health care facility (HCF) or electrical metallic tubing (EMT). Electrical boxes and bushings should be metal. 240 V cables have two 120 V hot conductors of opposite polarity, thus creating cancellation of electric fields without the need for special cable.

Order a Remote Shut-off

Order a product called a remote shut-off switch. A supplier is Safe Living Technologies. The product allows a remote control to shut off up to four circuit breakers. A box is installed next to the fuse box. The circuits connected should include those servicing bedrooms and rooms next to, over, and under bedrooms. The remote can be used to shut the power to the bedrooms off at night.

What Your Builder Should Know

Pools and Wells

Obtain the necessary permits to power a pool or a well with their own service panels. These should not be sub-panels from the house. An insulation union (section of plastic pipe or a dielectric union) should be inserted between metal pipes that go between the house and a pool, well, or equipment room serviced by separate main electric panels.

Water Pipes

If the water pipes are copper, they are not to touch the concrete. Run metal pipes through a piece of PVC as they penetrate the slab.

Concrete Reinforcement

Rebar is not permitted. If reinforcement is required, add fiberglass or polypropylene fibers such as Fibermesh 650 or Novomesh® 850/950 to the concrete mix.

Wiring Installation

Walls, ceilings, and floors around bedrooms should be free of wiring that serves high-current appliances, such as water heaters, freezers, boilers, stoves, ovens, and refrigerators.

Specifications for Reducing EMFs

Grounding and Bonding

Provide a separate grounding rod for each the phone and cable coaxial. Do not bond the phone or coaxial cable grounds to the ground used by the electric company.

Wiring Connections

Wires should be paired and balanced. The following are recommended to prevent errors that cause an unbalanced current:

- All wiring in an electrical box must be of the same circuit.
- No wiring of ½ switch outlets using different breakers.
- Four wire cable shall be used to wire three-way switches.
- The bare copper ground wires in each outlet box shall be insulated with spaghetti tubing and connected together with a wire nut or an insulated crimp connector to prevent inadvertent contact of ground wires with the neutral screws on outlets.
- 120 V appliances shall not be connected to a two-wire 240 V cable that uses the ground as the neutral.
- A dielectric union shall be installed on metallic gas and water lines in contact with an appliance such as a water heater, a boiler, or stove.

What Your Builder Should Know

Communications

Hard-wire the home for internet using ethernet cable. Hard-wire the house for stereo speakers.

Lighting

There shall not be florescent bulbs, LED bulbs, dimmer switches, or lighting that requires a low-voltage transformer.

Kill Switches

Light switches shall be installed to turn the power on and off for the dishwasher, microwave oven, and locations where a flat panel TV might be.

Specifications for Ventilation

Ventilators

A ventilator shall be installed to bring in fresh air and exhaust stale air independent of the central air-conditioning and heating system. A ventilator with dedicated ductwork shall be installed for each air-conditioning and heating system.

A supply vent should be installed in each bedroom and sitting area where there is an air-conditioning and heating supply vent.

A return vent should be installed in each room where a supply vent is installed. The return should be at the opposite end of the room, a minimum of 10 feet from the supply vent.

For rooms with a supply but no return vent, a return air pathway register shall be installed in the wall between the room and the hallway where the central return is located. These dampen sound and light transmissions (provide privacy) while allowing air to flow from one side of the wall to the other.

The exhaust for the ventilator should be on the roof and not close to (a least two feet from) sewer and plumbing vents.

The fresh-air intake should be on the side of the house, two to three feet below the roofline, and away from a dryer vent, kitchen range exhaust, gas meter, and garbage cans.

Exhaust Fans

Exhaust fans shall be quiet, less than 1.0 sone.

Make-up Air for Kitchen Range

An outdoor air intake shall be installed in the kitchen. Example products are the Broan SmartSense® Fan Automatic Make-Up Air Damper and products by CCB Innovations. It should be wired to open the damper on the outdoor vent when the hood is turned on. The vent should come through an exterior wall, pass under a kitchen cabinet, and terminate at a kick plate on one side of the stove. The intention is the outdoor air will not compete with gases exhausted from cooking. The outdoor air should mix with ambient air before being pulled into the exhaust.

Specifications for Ventilation

Make-up Air for Laundry Room

An outdoor air intake shall be installed in the laundry room to prevent the air pressure in the laundry room from becoming negative (less than outside) when the dryer is turned on. Examples are the Fresh Air Ventilation System and Control made by Honeywell, and products by CCB Innovations. It should be wired to open the damper on the outdoor vent when the dryer is turned on.

Exhaust Fan in the Garage

An exhaust fan shall be installed in the garage with a minimum of 80 CFM. It should run 24/7. The switch should be labeled with instructions to leave it on. Three-car garages should have two fans installed.

What Your Builder Should Know

Specifications for Minimizing VOCs

Termite Treatment

Do not apply a treatment for termites unless approved by the owner.

Concrete Forms

The use of petroleum-based form oils is prohibited. The following are acceptable: vegetable oil, an acceptable paint, BioForm™, Crete-Lease® (soy-based), or DUOG-ARD® (water-based).

Odor Barriers

Before the slab is poured, after the vapor barrier is installed, use the sealant tape for the vapor barrier to seal around pipes and electrical conduits that penetrate the slab.

After the slab is dry, seal the expansion joints and penetrations around plumbing, water pipes, and electrical conduits with silicone caulk.

Clean Metals

If the ductwork is sheet metal, the metal should be cleaned using a high-pressure hose and an approved cleaner, such as T.S.P., before the ducts are fabricated.

Ventilation

Install a ventilation system following the Specifications for Ventilation.

Exterior Sheathing and Subfloors

The following are unacceptable: OSB, products containing asphalt, paper-faced drywall, foam insulation board, and pressure-treated plywood.

The following are acceptable: CDX plywood, exterior grade plywood, AdvanTech™ plywood.

Insulation

Blown-in cellulose or mineral wool batts should be used for insulation. For cellulose, the installer shall use a hose 1 1/2 to 2 inches in diameter and install a density of 3 1/2 to 4 pounds per cubic foot of cellulose. The installer shall save the used bags to check that the project is in the ballpark in terms of the density of the insulation installed.

Specs for Minimizing VOCs

For mineral wool, Thermafiber® by Owens Corning is formaldehyde-free. The UltraBatt™ version is denser and easier to install.

In roofs with gables, baffles shall be installed to prevent insulation from blocking air flowing through soffit vents.

Grout Sealers

Sealers containing petroleum and solvents are prohibited. The following are acceptable: AFM Safecoat® Grout Sealer; AFM Safecoat® Safe Seal, which may be diluted 50:50 with water and mixed into dry grout; and sodium silicate (water glass), a clear liquid sealer that can be painted over grout.

Air Barrier

An air barrier shall be constructed between the garage and rooms next to and above the garage as follows:

- Install foam sealant tape under sill plates as the walls are being framed.
- After drywall is installed, use foam tape to seal between the bottom of the drywall and the floor.
- Use spray foam to seal around plumbing pipes and electrical wires going into walls.
- Use sealed can lights for recessed lighting.
- Before installing electric boxes, cover the backs with the fiberglass mesh used for drywall patching, and

paint over the mesh with a water-based duct mastic.

- After drywall is installed, caulk around electrical boxes between the boxes and drywall using an approved caulk.
- Install gaskets on light switch plates and electrical outlets.
- Caulk between the bottom of the door threshold and the slab.
- The door between the house and garage should be weather-stripped.

Paint

Use products GREENGUARD Gold certified or substitutes approved by the owner.

Spills shall be reported, noted where they occur, and cleaned up using approved cleaning products.

Plaster

Unacceptable plaster sealers include urethane and beeswax. Plaster shall be finished using a traditional white wash or an approved water-based sealer. The following are acceptable: MexeSeal by AFM Safecoat® (matte finish), Polyureseal BP by Safecoat® (gloss finish), and OKON® W-2 Water-Repellant Sealer. OKON has an odor. Test it on a scrap of plaster to make sure it is not objectionable.

Specs for Minimizing VOCs

Appliances

Water heaters shall be electric, on-demand.

Gas water heaters, if required, shall be on-demand, sealed combustion, power-vented outside.

Gas appliances, gas pipefittings, and connections shall be checked for leaks using a combustible gas sniffer. Flex hoses that leak shall be replaced, not tightened.

Gas appliances shall be tested for carbon monoxide. A probe shall be inserted into the flue or exhaust of each appliance. If a level greater than 100 ppm is measured, the appliance shall be repaired or replaced.

Gas ovens should be tested at the stovetop and inside the oven. The orifice for an oven should be adjusted or replaced to reduce the amount of carbon monoxide produced to less than 100 ppm. If a level of less than 100 ppm cannot be achieved, the stove/oven shall be replaced.

Chimney Draft-induction Fans

A draft inducer fan should be installed on top of chimneys.

Bathtubs

Before closing the wall behind a bathtub with drywall, cover any exposed soil around plumbing pipes with concrete, mortar, or plaster.

Finish Carpentry Wood

Solid wood should be used for applications such as shelves in closets and pantries.

Wood for finish carpentry should be formaldehyde-free.

If composite wood materials are required, use ultra low emission formaldehyde (ULEF) or no added formaldehyde (NAF) products.

Specifications for
Reducing Dust

Site Maintenance

The site, including sidewalks, the driveway, parking, the building entrance, and street, shall be kept clean and free of debris.

Smoking on the premise is prohibited, including outside and in the garage.

Maintain a waste container with a lid.

All waste must be removed from the house and the garage at the end of each day. This includes personal trash and material waste.

The floors should be vacuumed at the end of each day. This includes the garage.

Protection of Installed Work

If the cabinets arrive early, seal them with plastic and store them in a clean, dry location. Cabinets should not be installed until the drywall and painting are completed. Cover cabinets with polyethylene plastic and temporary tape after they are installed.

HVAC Systems

HVAC systems and ducts should not be placed in attics, a crawlspace, or garage.

The HVAC vents and return openings should be sealed during construction and not used for heating or cooling during construction.

HVAC Blower Compartments

Fiberglass and other materials used for insulation and acoustics inside the blower compartment shall be covered with foil and foil tape.

HVAC Ducts

Wall cavities and building plenums shall not be used as air ducts, including where an HVAC unit attaches to the return vent.

Ductwork shall not be located in exterior walls or under concrete slabs.

Sheet metal should be used for ductwork. The insulation shall be on the OUTSIDE on the metal ducts. Fiberglass duct board and flex type ducts should not be used.

Specifications for Reducing Dust

Duct seams shall be sealed with water-based mastic.

A duct blaster inspection should be performed to pressure check the ductwork before closing walls and ceilings with insulation and drywall. Leaks should be identified, repaired, and sealed with mastic.

HEPA Filter

Install a Pure Air Systems model 600HS Plus. Connect it to the HVAC in bypass mode.

Wall Assemblies

Before installing the insulation, wall cavities shall be vacuumed.

Fiberglass batt insulation should not be used in interior wall cavities for soundproofing.

Cutting Pipe

Request plumbers cover the floor with a tarp where they will be cutting and gluing PVC pipe or to cut pipe outside where the ground is covered with a tarp.

Chimneys

A draft inducer fan should be installed on top of chimneys.

Specifications for Healthy Water

Test the Water

Obtain a copy of the city water quality test report.

If there is a well, order the test for ninety-four contaminants from National Testing Laboratories. Test for fecal coliform using a local laboratory. Send a sample to Radon.com to be tested for radon.

Water Filtration Equipment

After obtaining the water test results, contact Krudico (800) 211-1369 for suggestions on filters.

For city water, a whole-house carbon tank system should be installed to remove chlorine.

If there is a well, install a UV system on the main line coming from the well to kill bacteria.

A reverse osmosis (RO) filter should be installed under the kitchen sink for drinking water.

What Your Builder Should Know

Install other water filtration equipment as needed based on the water testing report. Bottled water is not regulated by the Safe Drinking Water Act. Some bottled waters contain fluoride, bacteria, and other contaminantes.

Contaminant	Removed by a Carbon Filter	Removed by Reverse Osmosis (98%)*	Comments
Chlorine by-products	X	X	Install a whole-house treatment tank.
Fluoride		X	Requires reverse osmosis.
Lead, Copper		X	Most filters with carbon also have one that removes lead and copper.
Arsenic		X	Liver, kidney, and bladder cancers.
Nitrates		X	Hazardous for infants. Reduces oxygen in blood.
Pesticides	Varies	X	
VOCs	X	X	
Radon	X	X	An issue when showering and running dishwasher if levels are high.
Uranium		X	*2% can be too much depending on the level. A whole-house tank system is required to remove high

Swimming Pool and Hot Tub Water Treatment

Bromine and chlorine are toxic. A copper and silver type sanitizer system is recommended. Lifeguard Purification Systems (813) 875-7777.

The proper pool water chemistry (pH and hardness) must be maintained. Use a non-chlorine product such as potassium permanganate for shock treatment.

Specifications for Soundproofing

Walls

Frame two separate walls, back to back, leaving a space between them. The walls must not touch. Stagger the studs on each wall twenty-four inches on center, so they are not in line. Caulk along the bottom of sill plates as the walls are framed.

Use 1/2" drywall on both sides. The joints in the panels should not be in line. Avoid mounting electrical boxes in the same stud cavity of each wall. Stager outlets one or two stud bays on opposite sides of the walls.

Wrap pipes inside the wall with an insulating material.

In between the walls, install insulation such as fiberboard made from recycled paper or wool matting. Cellulose has soundproofing properties and may be used. Do not use fiberglass or foam. Spray foam is not effective for reducing noise.

What Your Builder Should Know

Floors

AdvaTech™ claims their plywood squeaks less.

The simplest way to soundproof floors is to install cork strips between floor joists and the subfloor.

Another is a brick floor on top of the subfloor, a layer of soft board, and a top layer of tile in thinset.

An elaborate design has a tongue and groove wood subfloor on sound insulating strips, under which there is a false floor in-filled with brick. The combination of brick and fiberboard provides the maximum reduction in noise and vibration.

Windows

To dampen noise from outside, install windows with heavy glass or dual-pane storm windows.

Air-conditioners and Fans

Do not put a compressor for an air-conditioner outside of a bedroom or sitting area. Do not put the fan for a radon-mitigation system outside a bedroom or sitting area.

Doors

Use solid interior doors. When installing doors, caulk between the doorjambs and house framing.

Appendix

References to Give the Builder

Include a section in your specifications for drawings, references, standards, and codes. The applicable section is 01 40 00 Quality Requirements, subsection 01 42 00 References. Include the following as references:

Roofing, shower bladders, and window flashing

Best Practices Guide to Residential Construction: Materials, Finishes, and Details. Steven Bliss. Wiley & Sons, 2005.

Stucco

Best Practices Guide to Residential Construction: Materials, Finishes, and Details. Steven Bliss. Wiley & Sons, 2005.

Vapor barrier under the slab

ASTM E 1745-09 Standard Specification for Water Vapor Retarders used in Contact with Soil or Granular Fill under

What Your Builder Should Know

Concrete Slabs.

ASTM E 1643-09 Standard Practice for Selecting, Design, Installation and Inspection of Water Vapor Retarders Used in Contact with Earth or Granular Fill Under Concrete Slabs.

STONE VENEER
Installation Guide and Detailing Options for Compliance with ASTM C1780 For Adhered Manufactured Stone Veneer. The Masonry Veneer Manufacturers Association.

BASEMENTS AND CRAWLSPACES
Builder's Guide. Available from the Energy Efficient Building Association or Building Science Corp.

MOLD REMEDIATION
IICRC S520 Standard Guide for Professional Mold Remediation.

WATER DAMAGE REMEDIATION
IICRC S500 Standard Guide for Professional Water Damage Restoration.

Cleaning Products

The following is an example of specifications for acceptable and non-acceptable cleaning products.

Prohibited cleaning products include:

Products that do not list all of the ingredients or have "other" or inert ingredients.

Products with the any of the following:

- antimicrobials
- fragrance
- chlorine, bleach, ammonia, or alcohol
- petroleum, phenol, glycol, or ethanol

Acceptable cleaning products include:

- fragrance-free dish soap
- white vinegar
- hydrogen peroxide
- borax
- baking soda and washing soda
- lemon juice

What Your Builder Should Know

Baking soda cleans, deodorizers, and scours. It is non-corrosive, slightly abrasive, and effective for light cleaning.

Borax cleans and deodorizes.

Hydrogen peroxide can be used as a substitute for chlorine bleach.

Hand or dish soap is an effective and gentle cleaner. Use fragrance-free.

T.S.P. substitute (trisodium phosphate substitute) works well for cleaning walls prior to painting. The normal T.S.P. is corrosive and requires rubber gloves. The substitute is phosphate-free and safer to handle.

Washing soda (sodium carbonate) cuts grease and removes stains. It's effective for laundry and general cleaning.

White vinegar cuts grease and removes lime deposits. An all-purpose cleaning solution can be made from white vinegar and plain water in a 50/50 ratio. For window cleaning, add 5 tablespoons of white vinegar to 2 cups of water in a spray bottle. A floor cleaner, excellent for ceramic tile, is made by mixing liquid dish soap with 1/4 quarter cup of vinegar and one gallon of water.

Lemon juice removes grease and sludge.

Cleaning Protocol

Cleaning should be done as work is in progress. The interior should be cleaned daily by vacuuming the floor, including the garage. Waste should be removed each day.

The following might be done as a final cleaning. You might think of a better way to do this and other times it should be done. These are the basic principles and suggested times for a deep cleaning in addition to daily housekeeping.

#1 The first cleaning is suggested after the house is framed BEFORE the sheathing (outside walls) are installed. A leaf blower should be used to blow dust off the framing, top to bottom, off the slab, and out of the house.

#2 The next cleaning is suggested BEFORE insulation is installed. The builder may schedule a framing walk-through the day before the insulation is installed. The house will have sheathing, doors, and windows. Use the leaf blower. As the house is closed up, you may want to follow the cleaning procedure in the next chapter. It makes use of a negative air machine to scrub the air and oscillating fans to keep the dust suspended. <u>This is a key moment to clean the house.</u> Once insulation is installed, dust in the wall cavities will be sealed inside them forever. Suggest the builder do this before the walk-through. The builder may have the insulation crew coming the same day the walk-through is completed.

#3 The next suggested cleaning is after the drywall is installed. Installing drywall creates a lot of dust (gypsum and silica) from cutting and finishing. Wait until the walls have been painted, otherwise the blower may blow dust off the unsealed finishes. This cleaning should be done before cabinets, carpet, and appliances are installed. Vacuum the floor of the big stuff before using the leaf blower. Use the negative air machines and oscillating fans as explained in the next chapter, the Cleaning Procedure.

Cleaning Procedure

Preparation

Seal the heating, ventilation, and air-conditioning ducts with plastic. Cover and seal cabinets. If the insides of the cabinets are dusty, use a compressed air hose to clean them out before covering them.

Open the windows.

Place air scrubbers in the middle of the main sections of the house (living room, hallway). If you rent air scrubbers, exhaust them outside by connecting ducts to their exhaust ports and running the ducts through a door or window to the outside. Do not use a rented scrubber without exhausting it outdoors.

Buy ten or more oscillating fans. Aim the fans randomly at the corners of rooms, walls, and ceilings. The purpose is to minimize stagnant air zones and to keep the dust suspended so it may be filtered out by the scrubbers and opened windows.

Use a Leaf Blower

Particles will fly out that could damage your eyes. Wear a full-face HEPA respirator or half-face HEPA respirator with goggles. A full-face HEPA respirator costs around $100; Half-faced HEPA respirators around $30. Wear earplugs.

Walk through the house with the leaf blower. Aim it at the corners of rooms, the floor, ceiling, walls, the tops of cabinets, steps, beams, fixtures, and doorjambs. It's a shotgun approach. Walk though waving it around. This should take no more than five minutes. Visible dust will result. Go outside and wait fifteen minutes for the dust to settle.

Vacuum the Big Stuff

Vacuum the floor. This should be a quick vacuum to get the big stuff. The floor will become dirty again the next round.

Repeat

To be effective, the leaf blower must be used several times, vacuuming in between. Allocate a full day.

Reposition the Fans

Every two hours, reposition the fans to hit new corners.

Cleaning Procedure

Do a Final Cleaning

When it appears the leaf blower no longer blows dust out into the open, and the air does not become hazy, proceed to a final cleaning as follows:

Vacuum all horizontal surfaces—floors, stairs, tops of cabinets, and so forth.

After vacuuming, use plain soap and water to damp-mop or damp-wipe all surfaces. Use non-fragrant dish soap. Work from top to bottom—ceiling, walls, tops of cabinets, floor. Use a ladder to reach tall walls and light fixtures.

If the furnace ducts or ventilation system were not covered during construction or got dirty, have the furnace and ventilation ducts cleaned by a professional. Do not use a sanitizer. You're cleaning, not trying to kill mold. Ask the duct cleaning company to use high-pressure air hoses and brushes and leave chemicals and sanitizers on the truck.

Additional References

Organic Indoor Air Pollutants. Occurrence, Measurement, Evaluation. Edited by Tunga Salthammer and Erick Uhd. Wiley-VCH, 2009.

Building Materials - Product Emission and Combustion Health Hazards. Kathleen Hess-Kosa. CRC Press, 2017.

Buildings Don't Lie, Better Buildings by Understanding Basic Building Science. Henry Gifford. Energy Saving Press, 2017.

Construction Specifications Writing, Principles and Procedures. Rosen, Kalin, Weygant, and Regener. John Wiley & Sons Inc., 2010.

What Your Builder Should Know

About the Author

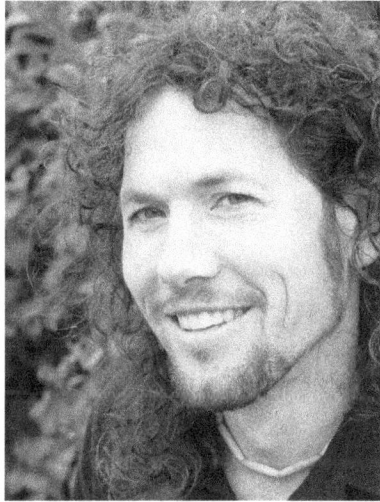

Photo by John Mate

Dan Stih is an aerospace engineer and consultant who investigates homes and offices to solve complaints and health problems related to being indoors. He got started after retiring as an engineer from Motorola and working as a handyman. While working as a handyman he discovered some clients who were sick had things wrong with the buildings they lived in, making it difficult for them to become well again.

Visit healthylivingspaces.com.